# Geriatric Medicine for Students

P9-AOF-926

McMASTER
Bookstore
12.20

## J.C. BROCKLEHURST

M.D. (Glas.), M.Sc. (Manc.), F.R.C.P. (Glas. & Edin.)

Professor of Geriatric Medicine,
University of Manchester


## T. HANLEY

M.D. (Lond.), F.R.C.P. (Lond.)

Consultant Physician in Geriatric Medicine
Harrogate District; Formerly Senior Lecturer in
Geriatric Medicine,
University of Manchester

# Geriatric Medicine for Students

J.C. BROCKLEHURST

T. HANLEY

Joseph A. Carvelli

CHURCHILL LIVINGSTONE
Edinburgh London and New York 1976

CHURCHILL LIVINGSTONE

Medical Division of Longman Group Limited

Distributed in the United States of America by Longman Inc.,
19 West 44th Street, New York, N.Y. 10036 and by
associated companies, branches and representatives
throughout the world.

© Longman Group Limited, 1976

All rights reserved. No part of this publication may be
reproduced, stored in a retrieval system, or transmitted in any
form or by any means, electronic, mechanical, photocopying,
recording or otherwise, without the prior permission
of the publishers (Churchill Livingstone,
23 Ravelston Terrace, Edinburgh EH4 3TL).

First Edition 1976
    Reprinted 1978

ISBN 0 443 01470 1

**Library of Congress Cataloging in Publication Data**
Brocklehurst, John C.
    Geriatric medicine for students.

    Includes index.
    1. Geriatrics. I. Hanley, Thomas, joint author.
II. Title. [DNLM: 1. Geriatrics. WT100 B864g]
RC952.B74    618.9'7    76–8473

Printed in Hong Kong by
Sheck Wah Tong Printing Press Ltd.

# Preface

Geriatric Medicine—the medicine of old age—stands as a discipline in its own right because it brings together four separate and unique elements. These are: the study of aging; the basic clinical problems of the elderly (falls, incontinence, mental confusion, etc.); the special features of disease in old age, and the organization and provision of medical, social and voluntary services for old people. Added to this is the fact that old people form the largest single consumer group of the medical and social services now, and will do so to an even greater extent at the end of the century.

These are the reasons why Geriatric Medicine must have its due place in the medical curriculum and these are the basic reasons for publishing this book.

This is a students' handbook, written particularly for medical students, but we hope it will also be seen as highly relevant to students in the professions ancillary to medicine and to student nurses. Even postgraduate students may find here material relevant to their studies, presented sufficiently broadly to give them a clear perspective of the practice of medicine in old age.

We are grateful to many people who have assisted in the production of this book, but we must thank especially Susan Williamson, who bore the major share of preparing the manuscript, and Brian Pearson and Keith Harrison, who prepared the diagrams.

We acknowledge also our thanks to the Editors of the *Lancet* and *Gerontologia Clinica* and to Dr MacMillan and his colleagues for permission to publish the figures.

Manchester,                                                J.C. Brocklehurst
1976                                                       T. Hanley

# Contents

# Part One: Aging and Old Age

# 1. Theories on the Nature of Aging

'What is aging, and what is its cause?' are questions that have long fascinated men (and women); the preoccupation is understandable, since human beings are the only living creatures capable of grasping aging as an idea and consequently of fearing it. Other animals accept in blissful unawareness only the physical actuality of the moment that is now.

One thing is certain —there is no single 'cause of aging', just as there never was a Philosopher's Stone nor an 'Elixir of Life'. Aging is multiform and though death is the inevitable end result of aging, it seems likely that it is an incidental effect, in the sense that it will occur when the aging processes happen to impinge on something, however small, which is vital for survival of the organism—the cells of the respiratory centre in Man for example. Keats' poetic view that 'death is life's high meed' makes no scientific sense.

*A machine analogy of aging.* The human organism can be legitimately regarded as simply one kind of machine, awesome in its complexity and durability but nevertheless a machine, doomed to suffer the fate of all machines which are regularly used. Sooner or later they develop faults, wear out and eventually cease to function, unless there is a minimal programme of servicing and replacement.

Pursuing this analogy, one can deduce some principles that might apply to biological aging:

1. Deterioration of a machine that is at all complex will occur at several different levels of organization. There is, at the lowest level, an inevitable deterioration with passing time of the basic materials, e.g. metal fatigue, wood decay and so on. At a higher level of organization there could be a failure of some component with a specific function, e.g. the spark plug of an internal combustion engine. Or there could be failure of a system such as the electrical

3

supply which serves many components. These three kinds of machine aging would roughly correspond with three levels of human aging: in cells, in organs and in tissues (the blood, which supplies oxygen to all the organs is the archetype).

2. The more complex the machine, the greater is the likelihood that faults will in fact appear; they will be of different kinds, have various degrees of importance for function of the machine as a whole and will evolve at different rates.

In spite of the fact that aging is like truth, 'a many sided thing', it is rational to look for one or a few processes that could be the common denominator of aging.

It has to be admitted at the start that theories abound, facts are few, and very little is known with certainty, but it seems logical that the mechanisms of biological aging should involve the same special properties that distinguish living things from non-living objects. Two basic properties are: (1) the capacity to reproduce and (2) the ability to draw energy from the external environment and marshal its use in an orderly way. Both these unique abilities of living organisms depend on the *capacity to synthesise proteins:* the physical form of an individual is determined by his structural proteins, and the main components of the biochemical machinery concerned with energy production, the enzymes, are also proteins. Another unique and remarkable property of living tissue is that it has, within the nuclei of its cells, a message in code which gives exact instructions for the synthesis of all proteins in the body.

It is, therefore, not surprizing that almost all current theories of aging focus on this coded system of protein manufacture as the most likely place for the passage of time to exert its effect. But within this general framework there are two quite sharply separated schools of thought, which believe that aging is caused by either:

1. Deterioration of the protein synthesising machinery
2. The continued operation of a programme which starts with embryonic development, continues as growth and differentiation, and terminates as senescence: an idea neatly described as the 'molecular clock' hypothesis.

## Aging theories based on deterioration of the protein synthesizing mechanism

The process of protein synthesis is distilled in a phrase as succinct as it is rhythmic:

### DNA makes RNA and RNA makes protein

Two main sub-theories of aging concern these individual steps. That based on abnormalities of 'DNA making RNA' is commonly called the 'primary error hypothesis' and that concerned with 'RNA making protein' is called 'non-DNA error theory'.

In order to understand these ideas it is necessary to grasp the bare bones of the coded system itself. The coded message giving instructions for protein synthesis is written along the length of one strand of the double helix of deoxyribonucleic acid ('DNA') contained in the cell nucleus. The 'letters' of the code are the special surface shapes of four substances: adenine ('A'), cytosine ('C'), guanine ('G') and thymine ('T'). For general comprehension, details of the chemistry are not important and we can refer simply to a DNA code alphabet of only four letters: A, C, G and T. The coded message consists of the particular sequence of these 'letters', just as a Morse code message is a two item code of dots and dashes which can be decoded into words.

The message, as noted above, is on only one strand of DNA: this single strand has to be made available by unwinding of the double helix, and it has to be unbroken to be perfectly comprehensible when decoded.

## Theories based on disturbances of 'DNA makes RNA'

Most primary error theories are concerned with the possible ways in which the coded information on DNA could be distorted:

1. Deformation of the 'letters' themselves: the 'free radical' theory suggests that oxidative changes in DNA makes some of the letters of the code unrecogniz-able. The evidence for this comes from the hastening of aging by radiation and by the effects of certain chemicals

which induce mutations. The attraction of the theory lies in the fact that anti-oxidants exist which protect against radiation effect: these disturbances offer at least a possibility of verifying the theory experimentally and there is some evidence that, in huge doses, aging may be slowed. The difficulty of the theory lies in finding the likely source of either intrinsic or extrinsic DNA damage in natural aging. The most universal, 'natural' source of mutation is cosmic ionizing radiation. The effect would be expected to consist of a series of random 'hits' affecting one cell at a time and producing different DNA abnormalities in each nucleus which is hit, but calculation of the probability of hits on DNA from this source makes it highly unlikely that extrinsically induced mutation is a significant factor in aging. Nor could the prevalence of genetic abnormalities in man be accounted for by known extrinsic factors.

2. Cross-linkage in macromolecules (DNA). The simplest example of this is in natural rubber, where loss of plasticity is associated with the development of cross-links between long, straight hydrocarbon chains. There is also extensive information on the occurrence of increased cross-linking of the chains in collagen (the main constituent of tendons) as age advances. This has come to be widely regarded as the central disturbance in the aging of connective tissue, though there is strong evidence that it simply implies maturity of collagen and not true aging. The idea that cross-linking in DNA could impede effective use of its coded information has been much speculated on, but solid fact is lacking, largely due to the immense technical difficulty involved in comparing 'young' with 'old' DNA.

3. Irreparable breakages in the DNA information strand are another possibility, but again without direct proof.

4. Changed capacity of DNA to react with histones, basic proteins which can 'cover' parts of the code, has also been suggested as an aging mechanism.

*Auto-immunity in relation to aging*
This theory, which is a special sub-theory based on DNA

mutation, proposes that the lymphocytes, the wandering cells which keep up a vigilant surveillance of what is 'self' and what is not, are also capable of somatic mutation and that this will modify their antigenic properties. The result could be widespread antigen/antibody reaction in different tissues: proponents of this hypothesis suggest that aging effects will be shewn by cumulative low grade histoincompatibility reactions in many tissues. One piece of indirect evidence for this is the increasing prevalence of various types of autoantibodies in elderly people.

## Theories based on disturbance of 'RNA makes protein'

To comprehend these ideas, it is necessary to understand how the genetic message is put to practical use. The DNA letters 'A' and 'T' can behave like 'lock and key', i.e. are complementary; so are 'C' and 'G', but no other pairs are possible. The 'lock and key' effect depends on a strict stereochemical fit of the two molecules.

The first step in decoding is to prepare a 'complementary' copy of the DNA message as a long chain of ribose-nucleic acid (RNA) in which 'U' replaces 'T'. The process is called 'transcription' and the transcribed copy is 'messenger RNA', a large molecule located in the cell sap at special assembly points called ribosomes.

*Example:*   DNA message:    C G A | T G G | C C T |
Transcribed on
'messenger RNA': G C U | A C C | G G A |

*Three basic facts*
*The code is in triplets:* each triplet specifies one particular
amino acid
*It is read in one particular direction*
*The starting point for reading out must be identified*

In the hypothetical example given above, the triplets are:

start here ⟶
read this way
| G C U | A C C | G G A | . . .

and the message now reads: 'assemble in turn the amino acids arginine, tryptophan, proline'.

Each amino acid concerned is carried to the construction site on small 'transport RNA' molecules specially designed to carry that particular amino acid. The transport RNA for a particular amino acid (there can be more than one) has a complementary 'anticodon' which keys into the messenger RNA 'lock' and so locates the amino acid when its code comes up on messenger RNA. The process can be visualized in Figure 1.

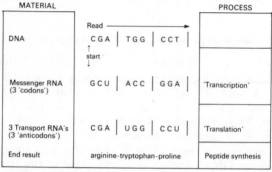

Fig. 1.1 The function of DNA/RNA.

This is an extremely simplified version of the process as to both detail and scale: a 'small' protein will contain about 300 amino acid units.

### The 'random error' hypothesis

Much attention has been paid to the possibility of random error in the transcription and translation processes described above. A particular hypothesis—the 'error catastrophe' hypothesis of Orgel—proposes that errors occur in the machinery for making enzymes, and more especially in those enzymes (polymerases) which are themselves involved in transcribing DNA: transcription by a faulty enzyme would be expected to increase errors further and set the scene for a self-accelerating effect culminating in a 'catastrophe'.

Medvedev has speculated that those structural genes which are expressed only once are more vulnerable to random error deterioration than the oft-repeated genes: the life spans of different species could conceivably be dependent on the species-specific ratio of unique to repeated genes (shortening as the ratio increases). Some of the chance errors which could occur in the course of transcription are:

1. deletions of one or more code letters
2. insertions of one or more code letters
3. insertions + deletions combined.

*The chemical consequence* of transcription errors is that a wrong sequence of amino acids is assembled after the error. An important point here is that all the possible 3-letter combinations of the 4 alphabet letters ($4 \times 4 \times 4 = 64$) are actually used. Some of the 20 possible amino acids have up to six codons, others have only one, and a few codons are used to indicate 'start', 'stop' or 'nonsense'. If a wrong 3-letter codon comes up on messenger RNA a 'wrong' amino acid will probably be fitted in, though there are certain built-in safeguards to suppress 'nonsense' messages. The length of the message that is wrong will depend on which particular coding errors have occurred (see Fig. 1.2).

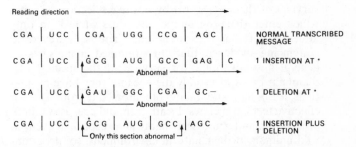

Fig. 1.2 The effect of various errors in messenger RNA.

The *physiological consequences* depend on whether or not any of the wrong amino acid sequences occur in those parts of the protein with functional importance, e.g. in the active centre of an enzyme.

Figure 1.2 (a hypothetical example) indicates the effects of various errors in messenger RNA.

The reader can test for himself the effect of other combinations such as three deletions, three insertions, a 'wrong start on the reading frame', etc. and draw general conclusions about the consequences of these.

## Theories based on 'molecular clock'

What has been discussed above is the effect of errors in the machinery itself, on the shop floor as it were. But it has also been suggested that one factor in aging might be changes in the 'management information' contained in DNA. In brief, 'management' is achieved by substances, probably basic histone proteins, which by the extent to which they 'cover' DNA decide whether or not the activity of a particular structure gene will be expressed. The process of growth and differentiation is a genetic programme in which certain genes are 'switched' on and then off in particular cells by 'molecular clocks' of some kind.

Within this general framework several quite distinct ideas are found:

1. That aging is simply a continuation of the 'programme' of differentiation, with death as the last item on it.
2. That aging has an evolutionary value for long-term survival of the species: (a) by positive selection of genes which enter the programme and are switched on only after maturity has been achieved. There is, however, no convincing evidence that 'programmed aging' has in general any advantage for survival of the species. Elephants in the wild usually die because they have ground their teeth flat, and many predators die from lack of effective teeth and claws. Death from old age, as we think of it in human terms, is probably an exceptional event in wild animals in their natural environment, so 'programmed senescence' could have relatively little selection value, since it is usually outpaced by other extrinsic causes of death

or

(b) by selection of genes which are an advantage in survival to maturity, but prove disadvantageous later, i.e. they would promote reproduction but ensure death.

Two other experimental findings are important in relation to the 'molecular clock' hypothesis: the 'transformation' of cell cultures, normally capable of only a limited span, to immortal cells, when they are infected by certain kinds of RNA (e.g. the Rous sarcoma virus and Rauscher mouse leukaemia virus). The normal sequence of events is: 'DNA makes RNA and RNA makes protein'. However, there is evidence that the reverse transcription 'RNA makes DNA' is possible in such infected cells: the abnormal DNA so produced could usurp the cells' normal genetic programme and would not be subject to the restraints that 'aging genes' would presumably apply to the cell's normal DNA.

The other finding is the 'Hayflick phenomenon': human embryonic lung fibroblasts grown in culture are capable of only about 50 doublings, after which they die. Cells taken from adult lungs die after fewer doublings—for each 10 years of chronological age one doubling is lost. This finding could be explained by a 'molecular clock' capable of counting nuclear doublings (the clock could not have simply counted elapsed time, because the fibroblast cultures could be held for long periods in the frozen state midway in the experiment; when unfrozen they resumed their doubling behaviour as though nothing had happened). However, the cells show chromosomal abnormalities at the end of their doubling period and the span could be limited by accumulation of errors in DNA.

All the preceding emphasis has been laid on the cell itself. But there is evidence that the medium in which cells exist can also influence age: some examples are known where tissue transplanted from aged animals to its normal state in young animals has resumed a lost function.

FURTHER READING

Brocklehurst, J.C. (1973) *Textbook of Geriatric Medicine and Gerontology.* Chapters by Rowlatt, C. and Franks, L.M., and by Hall, D.A. Edinburgh: Churchill Livingstone.

Comfort, A. (1964) *Ageing: The Biology of Senescence.* London: Routledge & Kegan Paul.

# 2. Sociological and Psychological Gerontology

Sociologists and psychologists both have contributions to make to the study of aging and many people from both disciplines now work exclusively in the gerontological field. The sociologist is concerned first with defining and describing the aging population, and secondly in considering the problems which an aging society poses, and the possible solutions to these. Psychologists on the other hand approach aging in three ways: firstly in developing tests of mental and intellectual function which may be used to measure the effects of aging on these functions; secondly to consider the experience of old people themselves, their desires and their problems, and thirdly to consider the attitudes of the rest of society towards old people and the reasons for these attitudes.

## Social gerontology

Every society approaches aging in its own way, but in advanced societies there is a good deal of common ground both

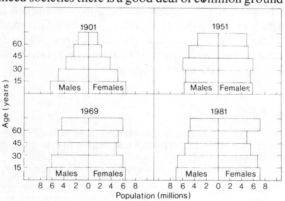

Fig. 2.1 Population of the United Kingdom (in millions) in the twentieth century.

12

in problems and the solutions. Population trends in the United Kingdom throughout the present century are well illustrated in Figure 2.1. Here we see that in the year 1900 our society was structured as a pyramid as far as age groups are concerned, with those in the first 15 years of life being by far the largest numerically. This picture has gradually changed to become first square and now, indeed, it is beginning to assume, at least as far as women are concerned, the appearance of an hour glass. These figures are reflected in those for life expectancy which are shown in Table 2.1.

Table 2.1  Life expectancy

|  | 1901 | 1971 | Increase (%) |
|---|---|---|---|
| *At birth* | | | |
| Male | 48·1 | 68·6 | 43 |
| Female | 57·8 | 74·9 | 45 |
| *At age 65* | | | |
| Male | 10·8 | 12·0 | 11 |
| Female | 11·9 | 15·9 | 34 |

There are two important reasons for this change: first the improvement in hygiene and nutrition in society, together with an increase in use of methods of birth control and secondly and more importantly the conquest of infectious disease. This has involved vaccination and inoculation, chemotherapy and, above all, the antibiotics. Whereas tuberculosis was the commonest cause of death in young adults at the beginning of this century, it is now a negligible cause of death at any age. Similarly, diseases such as diphtheria and the complications of measles and scarlet fever, of meningitis and of childbirth fever can no longer be regarded as of any real significance as major causes of death in our society. As a result, most people now survive into the years of retirement and the indications are that as time goes by we shall all live for ever longer periods of our life in retirement.

While the years of retirement are often regarded as being synonymous with old age, this of course is not the case and it is mainly beyond the age of 75 and particularly of 85 that the frailty and dependency of chronic illness and of age become apparent. It is salutary therefore to consider the changes we may expect in the different age groups in this country in the 20 years from 1971 to 1991 (see Table 2.2).

Table 2.2  Population projections (from the Office of Population Censuses and Surveys). Figures are in thousands.

| Population U.K. | 1971 | 1991 | Increase (%) |
|---|---|---|---|
| All ages | 55 668 | 60 263 | 8·25 |
| 65 + | 7 203 | 8 351 | 15·94 |
| 75 + | 2 522 | 3 464 | 37·35 |
| 85 + | 465 | 662 | 42·37 |

Apart from the obvious implication that retirement and old age are going to be the common experience of all of us in the future the most important economic consideration is the fact that the very old are the major consumers of social and medical services. At the present time our population includes two persons who are either below school leaving age or retired, to every three adults in the working population.

*Where retired people live*

Table 2.3 shows the type of accommodation occupied by the

Table 2.3  Accommodation of people aged 65 and over in England and Wales (1963)

| | | |
|---|---|---|
| Private households | 94·0% | 95·5% |
| Hotels, boarding houses, lodging houses | 1·5% | |
| Residential homes | 1·7% | |
| Psychiatric hospitals, nursing homes | 1·0% | 4·5% |
| Other hospitals and nursing homes | 1·8% | |

over-65's in a survey carried out in 1961. Over 95 per cent of the elderly population live in private houses (either their own, with relatives or friends) or in hotels and boarding houses and only 4·5 per cent live in institutions either residential or hospital. This latter number includes 1·0 per cent in mental hospitals, 1·7 per cent in old people's residential homes.

It is interesting that this figure of 4·5 per cent is lower than in other advanced societies. A cross-national survey comparing the UK with Denmark and the USA showed the following proportion of retired people living in institutions:

United Kingdom              4·5%
United States of America   4·6%
Denmark                    7·0%

This ranking in the international scales may have two implications. In the first place there is little doubt that most
elderly people would prefer to live independently in the community for as long as they possibly can and that any form of
institutional care is the last thing that they would wish for or
indeed should be encouraged to wish for. On the other hand
there is no doubt at all that a proportion of younger members
of the population in the United Kingdom are suffering almost
intolerable stresses, mental and physical, in trying to cope with
aged disabled relatives, especially those who are mentally disordered. A demented old woman who hardly realizes what is
night and what is day, who turns on gas taps and forgets about
them, who is likely to wander out into the streets in the day
time and get lost, or into her grand-children's bedrooms at
night and frighten them, may well be more than any individual
person should have to try and cope with for months or years
on end. The stress which may be engendered in this situation
may indeed lead to breakdown involving not only the chief
carer of the mentally disordered old lady but of the whole
family and indeed of the marriage. In view of the extent of
dementia (see p. 61) it may be argued that the figure of 4·5
per cent institutionalized old people in Great Britain signifies
greater hardship in this way than is apparent in other countries.

*Family contacts*

Such researches as have been carried out to discover the
extent to which old people and their families may retain contact with each other, indicate that in Great Britain people who
have children retain a very close contact with them. Unfortunately most of the work on which these figures are based is
now about 20 years old, and there may have been some change
since then. About one fifth of the elderly population are
childless, but of those who have children the contact they
retain with them is illustrated in Table 2.4. Maintaining contact with children, of course, is not necessarily the same thing
as receiving companionship from them since it is possible for

Table 2.4  Family contacts of people aged 65 + (Townsend. 1955)

---

No surviving children: 20%

Of the remainder:
80% saw child daily
 4% saw child less than once weekly

52% lived in same dwelling
25% lived within 5 minutes' walk
 8% lived more than 5 minutes' walk but less than a mile

---

an elderly person to live in her son or daughter's house and be almost a stranger, confined to her own room with little contact with anyone else. However, this is exceptional and while very often old people will maintain their strong determination not to impose any load on their children by going to live with them, it seems to be the case that the majority of widows and widowers do in fact live in the same dwelling as one or other of their children.

Decisions concerning the future way of life, particularly either moving into a residential home or moving in to live with the family, should as far as possible never be taken at a time of crisis, such as immediately after a bereavement. The family physician should be able and willing to advise on these matters, even if he does no more than indicate the various possible pathways that are open and the risks and advantages of each.

*Loneliness*

It is often said that loneliness is the scourge of old age. Inevitably at a time when a spouse is lost and when other friends and contemporaries are dying and when this is associated also with increasing infirmity, perhaps limited mobility and with sensory deprivation (especially deafness), loneliness can only be expected to become more common than at earlier ages. It is important not to confuse loneliness with being alone. Many people live alone quite happily and others can be lonely in a crowd. There can be little doubt that loneliness is a real problem among elderly people and it is here that the voluntary organizations have more to offer perhaps than any other, in providing friendly visitors and a whole network of clubs and day centres, together with some assistance with transport to get there. The general practitioner should be fully aware of voluntary services that are available in his area and what they can provide. Indeed the complete family doctor will be prepared to stimulate the voluntary services to discover the gaps in their services and to attempt to fill these.

## Retirement migration

An important fact about elderly populations in Great Britain is that they are spread unevenly over the face of the country. For good or ill, people tend to retire to the holiday resorts and so areas like the South coast, the North Wales coast and the main holiday towns in the North West and North East of England have a resident population which is entirely unbalanced on an age basis compared to the rest of the country. Some figures are shown in Table 2.5. These figures imply

Table 2.5 Proportion of population of pensionable age in various towns.

| | |
|---|---|
| Total population (Great Britain) | 16·0% |
| Bexhill | 44·2% |
| Worthing | 38·8% |
| Clacton | 36·3% |
| Eastbourne | 33·4% |
| Colwyn Bay | 32·3% |
| Morecambe and Heysham | 31·4% |
| Torbay | 30·6% |
| Lytham St. Annes | 29·1% |
| Bournemouth | 28·1% |

much greater demand on social and medical services in the areas concerned and indeed on housing and other community services.

## The psychology of aging

Various psychological tests are the tools which psychologists use in carrying out their work. These are very important in relation to old age both in research and in the management of patients. Of the many tests which are used for this purpose, probably Wechsler's Adult Intelligence Scale is the best known. This is the special field of the psychologist and will not be dealt with in detail here. Such tests may indicate impairment of intellectual function and may give some indication also of the prognosis in relation to brain disease. They may be used in discovering the potential of old people to benefit from rehabilitation.

*Old people's attitudes towards aging*

Some psychologists have suggested that old people may have one of two attitudes towards aging:
1. Body transcending
2. Body preoccupation.

Leisure and comfort may mean predominantly physical well-being and to such a person the increase in frailty which accompanies age may be hard to bear. Others suffer severe pain and discomfort, but for them social and mental sources of pleasure and self-respect transcend those of discomfort. It is likely that these types of aging are extensions of such types of personality in younger life.

In general it seems that the very old living in the community form an élite, who are optimistic about health, seem to have a high social conscience and maintain high spirits. In fact it has been shown that most old people think their own health is at least as good as, if not better than, that of their contemporaries.

A strongly held tenet of psychological gerontology until about 10 years ago was the *theory of disengagement*. This theory suggested that the mutual withdrawal of society and of the individual from each other was a necessary condition for successful aging and for the proper functioning of society, and was the best thing that could happen both for the aging individual and also for society. Nowadays this theory has been generally superseded and there is reasonable confidence that for most old people the maintenance of a very high level of social involvement and activity is an important ingredient of successful aging. Indeed there is a welcome and increasing trend for old people to become involved in educational activity, widening their intellectual experience and exploring ideas which are quite new to them. Further education classes cater for them in a host of different ways. Some indeed are taking degree courses at the Open University.

It has been said that 'the normal, reasonable, well adjusted old person is fairly realistic in his appraisal of facts, accepts himself for what he is, tends to see his wife as an equal partner in a joint enterprise and is fairly tolerant in his assessments of the worth of his close relatives'.

*Psychological accompaniments of aging.* A number of age-associated factors which are measurable relate to the psychologist's view of aging. For instance, reaction time is slowed and in the face of this an old person in unable to retain both speed and accuracy. This is one of the reasons why older workers find it impossible to keep up with the pace of conveyor belts in manufacturing and is one of the biological reasons why retirement becomes a necessity for many people.

Another function affected by aging is *memory*. It seems that long-term memory, particularly memory of the very distant past, is retained throughout life. However as people age the ability to commit new material to memory diminishes and they seem, therefore, to dwell more and more in the past. Perhaps, these postulated changes in the function of memory are more apparent than real. Memory consists of committing new facts by a process of retention and this requires a number of other attributes. For instance, the desire must be strong enough to memorize the new material and this involves motivation. Once a career is passed this motivation may wane, as may drive. Similarly there must be a high degree of interest in the matter being committed to memory.

If memory tends to fail, for whatever reason, with advancing age, then the older person is at a disadvantage in a technological society where the experience which has been accumulated over a number of years may become obsolete and new techniques have got to be mastered.

The advantage which the old person has is in accumulated experience and in wisdom. These, however, are often less relevant in our type of society than in earlier and less sophisticated societies. One of the fruits of this is that some old people accept opportunities which only occur later in life, such as the writing of memoirs, textbooks, an interest in history and indeed an interest in old age itself. The older person of course may have an accumulated experience in the manipulation of society and a familiarity with its social machinery, such as committees, rules, rituals and other procedures. These are more likely to be of advantage in positions within the establishment than to workers in factories.

*Stereotypes of psychological aging.* One interesting psychological experiment involved the observation for various characteristics of a large elderly male population. By analysis of the scatter produced when these qualities were graphed, it was possible to identify stereotypes of aging. Perhaps the most striking thing is the way in which these stereotypes are in the main continuations of the individual's earlier life characteristics. Stereotypes were as follows:

1. *Constructiveness.* A well integrated man who enjoys life and its relationships, humorous, tolerant, flexible and self-aware, having had a happy childhood and continuity in life history.

*Aging.* He accepts the fact of old age, retirement and death, retains the capacity to enjoy (food, work, drink, play and sex), looks back with few regrets and looks forward to what is to come.

2. *Dependency.* Socially acceptable, but passive, unambitious person with fairly good insight. Tends to be over-optimistic and impractical. Married late and tends to be dominated by his wife.

*Aging.* Glad to retire, eats and drinks too much, gambles and enjoys holidays; has no enjoyment from such work as he may have to do.

3. *Defensiveness.* A person with a stable occupational history, well-adjusted and socially active, who has always planned ahead and refused help; emotionally somewhat over-controlled, conventional and habit bound; compulsively active.

*Aging.* Afraid of old age, puts off retirement, sees few advantages in it and ignores the prospect.

4. *Hostility.* This man tends to blame circumstances or other people for his failures. Complaining, aggressive, suspicious, he often has an unstable occupational history and incompetence in a number of minor ways.

*Aging.* Sees nothing good in old age, afraid of death, envies the young, plunges into active work to defer the evil day.

5. *Self Hate*. A person who is critical and contemptuous of himself, unambitious; a life marked by social and economic decline; unhappily married, with few hobbies; feels himself a victim of circumstances.

*Aging*. Accepts the facts of aging; not envious of the young, has had enough and looks for a blessed relief in death.

*Suicide*. It is an unfortunate fact that the suicide rate is higher among the elderly than among any other group of the population. Among the aged it is even higher among those living alone. It may be related to bereavement, loss of relations and friends and physical or psychiatric illness.

## Retirement

Retirement is such a crucial accompaniment of aging in western society that it requires careful consideration by doctors. The physician should understand something of the problems and implications of retirement, recognize it as a possible ingredient in a number of illnesses and be in a position to advise about how retirement should be approached.

Retirement is a new phenomenon inasmuch as in the second half of the twentieth century for the first time almost everyone is going to spend a significant number of years living in retirement. Retirement can, and indeed should, be a time of fulfilment when the elderly worker is at last released from toil which may not have been congenial and is free to enjoy the other things in life which he has not been able to devote much time to when he was working. This is the ideal picture and there is no doubt that for many people this is the actuality. More often than not, however, it is the person who has enjoyed his work who will also enjoy his retirement and he whose work has been a drudgery may well also find retirement a time of tedium.

Retirement is inevitably associated with a number of types of loss:

1. *Loss of finance*. Most people will be significantly poorer after retirement than before and those who depend on the State Retirement Pension will find that they have an

income which is at the present time less than one quarter of that of average male industrial earnings.

2. *Loss of status.* A man's position in the world is frequently judged by his work. Thus the day before he retires he may be the bank manager, the school teacher, the foreman in a factory, or a railway guard. The day after he retires he becomes an old age pensioner. This transition involves a considerable and usually unlooked-for change in status.

3. *Loss of companionship.* For most people their work is the place where they have most human contact. Indeed for the majority of people in our industrial society it is the principal social organization that they belong to. When they stop work they also lose this large element of companionship and social intercourse.

4. *Loss of orderly and purposeful occupation.* However much people may like or dislike their occupation there is no doubt that the routine which it involves is something by which most of them have come to live. This is perhaps the easiest thing to replace, but such replacement does not always happen.

These are probably the most important losses on retirement and perhaps their particular hazard is in the fact that generally they assail the pensioner without his really realizing what was going to happen to him and without his having taken any steps to prepare for it.

With the increased availability of leisure time and with increased education all round, people in the future will probably be better able to cope with the bonus years which retirement brings. However, it is likely that some form of preparation, five to ten years before retirement actually happens, will have a significant effect in preventing some of the medical and psychological problems of the retired.

This problem of pre-retirement training is being tackled by a number of education authorities and also by a voluntary body the Pre-Retirement Association (see p. 238). Doctors will be increasingly involved both in teaching on pre-retirement courses and also in general counselling in relation to retirement.

## Environment

Finally in considering social and psychological aging it is worth recording that environment inevitably contributes to the success or failure of this process. Physical design of the space in which elderly people live, the fact that they should be safe and secure without being segregated, that shops and public buildings should be easily accessible and indeed that shopkeepers and public servants should recognize the special needs of the old (particularly those living by themselves) are important. The elderly depend very much on public transport to maintain their mobility and yet vehicles seem to become all the time more hazardous for old people to use.

FURTHER READING

Bromley, D.B. (1974) *The Psychology of Human Ageing*, second edition. Harmondsworth: Penguin.

Townsend, P.B. (1963) *The Family Life of Old People*. Reprinted in 1970. Harmondsworth: Pelican.

Townsend, P.B. (1964) *The Last Refuge*. London: Routledge & Kegan Paul.

Tunstall, J. (1972) *Old and Alone*. London: Routledge & Kegan Paul.

Willmott, P. & Young, M. (1960) *Family and Class in a London Suburb*. Reprinted in 1968. London: Routledge & Kegan Paul.

# 3. Geriatric Patients

Old age is the period of life which makes greatest demands on medical services. The average number of consultations per year with general practitioners is 6·3 for the over 65's compared with 3·8 for the whole population. Forty per cent of hospital beds are occupied at any one time by people aged 65 and over, and it is predicted that this could rise to 80 per cent, by the year 2000. These facts stem from a number of important characteristics of disease in the elderly.

1. Some changes affect almost everybody who lives long enough and can therefore be regarded as changes due to aging and not due to disease.
2. There are the many chronic and disabling conditions which people accumulate in the course of their lives and which once acquired are never lost.
3. There are the precarious social circumstances of many old people.
4. Old people are more susceptible to acute illness than other groups of the population.

All these factors indicate both the human and the economic importance of dealing with illness in old people in a thorough and competent manner. It is sometimes argued that when people are approaching the end of their lives medical treatment is less relevant and investigation may therefore, be justifiably, less thorough. The very opposite, however, is the case because almost all disease processes can be ameliorated in elderly people and some can be cured. Unless the initial examination is thorough some important aspect of the spectrum of disability may be overlooked and the last years of an old person's life may be unnecessarily dependent on others. Because disease in old age is so complex and because its concomitant disabilities may so affect the life not only of the patient but of his family and of the society in which he lives there is every reason why medical examination and assessment should be just as meticulous at this age as at any other.

It is a truism that biological age and chronological age do not coincide: some people are old in their sixties and many are relatively young in their eighties and nineties. Too much attention, therefore, must not be paid to chronological age, although there are usually obvious differences between people in their sixties and those in their eighties. The late seventies would seem to mark the turning point into old age for most people nowadays.

A *geriatric patient* is characterized by the four factors mentioned above, and these will now be considered in more detail.

*First,* is the general background of age change which is bound to have some limiting effect on a number of body functions; perhaps the most obvious of these are *memory loss,* the effects of *presbyopia* (presbus = old man, ops = eye thus the visual changes associated with age) and of *presbyacusis* (akousis = hearing). Other bodily functions affected by age include posture (as old people get older they show an *increase in sway* when they stand upright) and *bladder function* (bladder capacity diminishes because of impairment of cerebral control of micturition).

It is not always easy to distinguish between the changes which are attributable to age and those which are attributable to disease. A good example of this is the condition of *osteoporosis* (particularly important because it predisposes to bone fracture). Osteoporosis is generally regarded as an age-associated disease of unknown cause. *Atherosclerosis* also is undoubtedly a disease process, although in the western world there are few who escape its effect as they grow old. Impairment of the *control of body temperature* and of the *maintenance of blood pressure* on change of posture are also common phenomena in the aged, and it is by no means certain whether these are always effects of cerebrovascular disease or whether they may in part be due to age changes in their controlling centres in the brain.

To these age changes which affect almost everybody as they grow older must be added the *second* factor, an accumulation of *degenerative* or chronic pathological conditions which, once acquired, remain for the rest of life. These include osteoarthrosis; disc degeneration and spondylosis; foot deformities; chronic lung disease; manifestations of arterial disease, such as myocardial ischaemia, cerebral ischaemia and infarction and peripheral vascular disease. Similiarly, chronic psychiatric disorders may accompany a patient into later life and add to the background of his disability.

*Thirdly*, and in addition to all those mentioned above, is the *social precariousness* in which many old people live. As a result of retirement and bereavement they may be isolated. Because of physical and mental disability they may be dependent on a whole range of social services including special arrangements for housing, domestic help, provision of meals, home nursing and many other services. Indeed, there is far more likely to be a link between social and medical problems in old people than in people of any other age group and neither may be dealt with in isolation.

*Fourthly*, and finally (as the straw that breaks the camel's back), there may be an incident of acute infection, infarction, trauma, haemorrhage, drug effect, or the sub-acute development of anaemia, metabolic disorder, etc.

## History and examination

Illness in old age is thus extremely complex. The history and clinical examination must therefore discover not only what is the final and precipitating factor which has actually brought the patient to his doctor, but also what are the other diagnoses and so, adding them all together, what is the nature of the total disability.

For practical purposes, indeeed, it is better to think in terms of *problems* then of diagnostic labels. The problems are those things which make it difficult for the old patient to live independently in the community. They are functional difficulties. A hemiplegia, for instance, may have very different implications as far as future life style is concerned for the elderly man living with his wife and for the aged spinster living entirely alone. While a full list of diagnoses should always be made at the end of the examination, the problems should also be listed.

History taking is often difficult because of deafness, dysphasia or mental disorder. It is advisable, if possible, to corroborate the patient's history with information from a relative or friend. In such a case, first take as full as history as possible from the patient and then while he is being prepared for examination the relative's version of the history should be obtained also.

If there is some doubt as to the reliability of the patient's story because of either loss of memory or clouding of consiousness, then *tests of memory and awareness* should be built into the history taking. It is usually possible to do this by asking the patient what he does all day and particularly whether or not he reads and if so which newspaper or magazine he reads or which was the last book he finished; whether he watches the television and if so which is his favourite programme; or about the news? Who is the Prime Minister? The Queen?: then by telling him quite directly that it is important to test his memory, and see if he can recall the names of five towns, five flowers, five colours. Finally, ask him if he is good at arithmetic and go on to a few simple tests such as 'serial sevens' (7 from 100, 7 from 93, 7 from 86, etc.,) counting the months of the year, forwards and then backwards and so on.

These tests can be introduced quite naturally and will allow the physician to evelute the accuracy of the information obtained in the history. In the history special note should always be made of evidence of dysuria: how many times the patient has to get up at night to empty his bladder; whether there is any incontinence and if so what is its nature. Ask also about falls in the previous year. If there have been any they must be described. It is often necessary to ask relatives whether there have been any episodes of mental confusion, abnormal behaviour, hallucinations etc.,.

Find out also about diet, particularly if the patient lives alone. Sometimes this is best discovered by asking him to recall what he has actually eaten in the last 24 or 48 hours. It is important to know what social services he is having, where his family is and whether they are seen regularly, when he retired, what was his work before he retired. At this stage it is possible to find out whether his 'spirits' are good or not, and whether or not he is lonely.

Before he lies down for the examination his gait should be examined and he should be examined for ataxia by asking him to stand with his feet together, first with his eyes open and then closed.

The *clinical examination* will be along the same lines as in a person of any age and will not be considered in detail here. A number of special factors which should be noted are dealt with in other parts of this book. A few general points in examination may be explained here.

The weight should be measured and since it is often not helpful to relate this to the actual height of an old person, an estimate of his height at maturity may be obtained by measuring the span of outstretched arms from finger tip to finger tip. Particular attention should be paid to muscle wasting, to the joints and feet, the tongue and teeth.

## Central nervous system

Power and co-ordination in the limbs may be rapidly estimated by having him perform three simple manoeuvres: first, stretch out his arms in front of him and see if he can maintain them in one position when his eyes are closed; secondly, he should tap the back of one hand quickly with the other hand repeating this manoeuvre for each hand, and thirdly perform the heel —knee test. If abnormalities are found they should be examined in more detail.

It is often difficult to estimate muscle tone in the elderly because of guarding around osteo-arthritic joints. An unusual type of increase in muscle tone in old people is *paratonic rigidity* (Gegenhalten) which is a manifestation of apraxia in patients with cerebral arterio-sclerosis (see p. 39). Deep reflexes may be diminished by age change in the peripheral nerves slowing conduction. In particular the ankle jerks are often lost. Sensation is usually retained apart from vibration sense which again is often lost in the legs.

In examining the central nervous system always estimate the visual fields, looking especially for homonymous hemianopia in patients with stroke.

## Cardiovascular system

Added heart sounds are often more significant than murmurs in heart disease in old age and should be carefully noted.

Rhythm disorders are also frequent. Blood pressure should be measured with the patient both lying and standing. To estimate postural hypotension the patient should stand for two minutes after having been lying down for five to fifteen minutes, and then the standing blood pressure measured. The presence or absence of peripheral pulses should always be noted.

*Respiratory system*

It is important to have the patient take a few deep breaths if crepitations are present at the lung bases, since these are sometimes due to poor respiratory excursion associated with immobility and they will then clear on deep breathing.

*Gastrointestinal system*

Within the abdomen the aorta of an old person is often prominent and hard, particularly in someone who is thin and has a tortuous and sclerotic aorta. It must not be confused with a tumour.

The soundness of the abdominal wall may be judged by having the patient lift his head off the pillow. The presence of palpable faeces should always be noted.

*Rectal examination* should never be omitted because constipation is such a common complaint in old age and in addition an unsuspected carcinoma of the rectum is occasionally diagnosed by this means. It is sometimes difficult to distinguish between hard faecal masses in the rectum and a carcinoma and if there is any doubt the examination should be repeated after emptying the rectum by an enema.

In patients with dysuric or vulvo–vaginal symptoms the vulva should always be examined, although a bimanual examination is often not required.

## Laboratory tests and special investigations

Because anaemia, hypokalaemia and bone disease are so common in old age a full blood count, biochemical profile and estimate of serum electrolytes should always be done at the initial examination. Urine analysis for protein and sugar should always be carried out, and if dysuric symptoms are present a mid-stream specimen of urine sent for culture. It is good practice in hospital consultation to obtain an ECG and a chest X-ray at the first examination. Even if these reveal no treatable abnormality they may still be important as base line information for the future.

Special investigations will be discussed in the text and these must always be undertaken if remediable pathology is suspected. It is often justifiable, and indeed important, to carry out tests to confirm a diagnosis even if the illness is not thought to be treatable. In planning the patient's future an accurate prognosis is needed and sometimes if these investigations are omitted because it is thought that the patient is too old, wrong diagnosis will be made which may seriously affect his management over a number of years.

Since old people are so prone to constipation special preparation is needed before sigmoidoscopy or barium enemas are carried out. Overnight admission to hospital is usually required in order to have a properly prepared patient and to save a lot of expensive professional time. Very often bowel preparation has to be carried out at home for several days beforehand as well.

In disease of the central nervous system the limits of investigation are sometimes more difficult to define. There need be no hesitation in using non-invasive techniques (e.g. brain scan and ultra-sound investigations). Angiography should only be undertaken if the patient is believed suitable for operation, should an operative lesion be discovered. More hazardous and uncomfortable procedures like air encephalography will not often be used in very old people.

# Part Two: Major Geriatric Problems

# 4. Cerebral Syndromes

Arterial disease is the greatest single cause of morbidity and disability in the elderly and its effects are seen particularly in three places: in the brain; in the heart and in the legs. In the brain, arterial disease may cause one of a number of well-recognized syndromes in the elderly, but may also lead to less clear-cut clinical changes. In addition, vascular changes may coexist with other pathological changes in the brain such as the senile plaques and neurofibrillary tangles of senile dementia which are discussed in Chapter 7. Another important factor is that cerebral arterial insufficiency may predispose to an acute confusional disorder which is then precipitated by some further impairment of the function of cortical neurones whose blood supply is already critically diminished. Thus superadded anoxia (due for instance to bronchopneumonia, hypotension as in myocardial infarction, or toxaemia, e.g. due to drugs or infection) may cause the temporary derangement of a brain which is already suffering from vascular insufficiency.

These are all important matters in considering the various cerebral syndromes in the elderly and help to account for their bewildering variety.

## Cerebral circulation

There are four pillars on which the whole circulation of blood to the brain rests—the two internal carotid arteries and two vertebral arteries. Their sources and courses are shown in the accompanying diagram (Fig. 4.1).

The common carotid artery arises from the innominate artery on the right and directly from the aorta on the left. It divides into the internal and external carotid and there is some anastomosis between these two through the ophthalmic artery

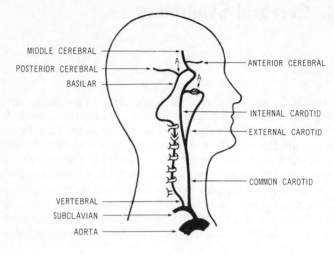

MIDDLE CEREBRAL
POSTERIOR CEREBRAL
BASILAR
ANTERIOR CEREBRAL
INTERNAL CAROTID
EXTERNAL CAROTID
COMMON CAROTID
VERTEBRAL
SUBCLAVIAN
AORTA
A = ANASTAMOSIS

Fig. 4.1 Cerebral circulation.

(where branches anastomose with branches of the frontal and lateral temporal arteries). The *internal carotid* finally passes through the carotid canal to enter the skull and then divides into the *anterior* and *middle cerebral arteries.*

The *vertebral arteries* arise from the subclavian artery and pass backwards to enter the foramina in the upper six cervical vertebrae. The position here is illustrated in Figures 4.2 and 4.3 from which it will be apparent that the vertebral arteries are susceptible to the effects of a number of pathological and aging processes affecting the neck.

After passing through the transverse processes of the atlas the vertebral arteries enter the skull through the foramen magnum. They lie on the dorsal part of the hindbrain coming together to form the *basilar artery* overlying the pons and after giving off the *posterior inferior cerebellar arteries* the basilar artery divides into the two *posterior cerebral arteries.*

The most important anastomotic device which ensures blood supply to the highly vulnerable cells of the brain, even if one of the four principal arteries is occluded, is the Circle of Willis, which is formed from the vessels already mentioned by

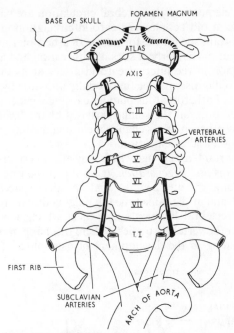

Fig. 4.2 The vertebral arteries.

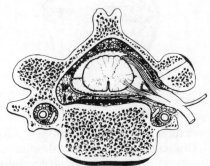

Fig. 4.3 Cross-section of a cervical vertebra showing the vertebral arteries within the vertebral canals.

an anterior communicating artery joining the two anterior cerebral arteries and by two posterior communicating arteries joining the middle and posterior cerebral arteries.

All the elements of the cerebral circulation are particularly vulnerable in old people. The carotid circulation in the neck is an important site for the formation of atheromatous plaques which occur particularly at sites of bifurcation and are especially common in the internal carotid artery at its origin. The Circle of Willis also may be functionally impaired by extensive formation of atheromatous plaques causing a general narrowing. In addition, all the smaller arteries of the brain may be affected by atheromatous change including medial fibrosis and hyalinization and calcification.

An important age change which may affect vertebro–basilar circulation is *disc degeneration*. It results in the intervertebral discs becoming 'squashed' so that the disc spaces become narrowed, and at the same time the bulging disc margins carry the inter-vertebral ligaments and their attached periosteum away from the vertebral bodies. Where this happens new bone forms, leading to the development of osteophytes (Fig. 4.4).

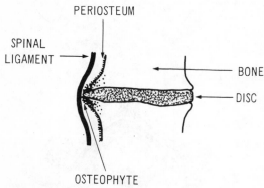

Fig. 4.4  Disc degeneration.

Disc degeneration is one of the reasons for loss of height with aging. This effect in the cervical spine is illustrated diagrammatically in Figure 4.5. It is generally known as *cervical spondylosis*.

For all these reasons the cerebral circulation in old people is at a critical level and its uneasy equilibrium may therefore be upset by super-added factors (anoxia, hypotension, toxaemia, focal vascular occlusions) which in a younger person with

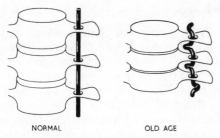

NORMAL          OLD AGE

Fig. 4.5  Changes in cervical spine as a result of disc degeneration.

a well functioning circulation would not cause any cerebral symptoms. This is one of the important reasons why mental confusion is such a common presenting symptom of the disease of the elderly.

## The old brain and vascular disease

In addition to episodic periods of vascular insufficiency referred to above, prolonged widespread impairment of cerebral circulation leads eventually to cerebral atrophy and a number of other characteristic pathological changes.

For instance the *état criblé* and *état lacunaire* may be seen by the naked eye as tiny, smooth walled cavities containing minute tortuous arteries. These are evident particularly in the basal ganglia and in the central white matter of the brain.

Another change affecting the tiny cerebral arteries is the formation of *micro-aneurysms* (first described by Charcot in 1868). These micro-aneurysms may be the seat of small haemorrhages or infarcts.

All of these changes, the états criblé and lacunaire and micro-aneurysms, become more common with advancing age and they also become more common in patients with hypertension. The hypertension may also cause haemorrhages and infarcts distributed with disparity near the white matter of the cerebral cortex. It is possible that microemboli from atheromatous plaques in the vessels in the neck also contribute gradually to cerebral cortical dysfunction. Finally there has been described also a congophilic angiopathy (i.e. amyloid formation) affecting the small arteries in the brains of about 15 per cent of old people.

## Clinical syndromes

In view of the widespread changes which may affect the aging brain and its blood supply it is not surprising that there is also a fairly large spectrum of clinical syndromes reflecting these changes and that there is a good deal of overlap between these. These conditions are particularly important in patients who have suffered from hypertension or in whom there is evidence of several overt cerebral infarcts. However, many of them may also exist without either of the above conditions being fulfilled. It is convenient to consider these syndromes in three groups:
1. Those affecting the whole brain
2. Those affecting predominantly the carotid territory
3. Those affecting predominantly the vertebro basilar territory.

## Cerebral arteriosclerosis

This is the general name for syndromes falling in the first category, that is affecting the whole brain. The clinical picture may contain one or more of three main elements:

Dementia

Apraxia with muscle rigidity and brisk tendon reflexes

Parkinsonism.

Arteriosclerotic dementia (see Ch. 7) is not always a feature of the syndrome of cerebral arteriosclerosis.

Parkinsonism is dealt with on page 47. Arteriosclerotic Parkinsonism is a clinical rather than a pathological entity. The common clinical features are rigidity, akinesia and loss of expression, whereas tremor, sialorrhoea and the other autonomic effects associated with paralysis agitans are not usually found. The Glabellar Tap sign is commonly positive.*

The basic syndrome of cerebral arteriosclerosis which may or may not have the other elements of dementia and Parkinsonism superadded are of apraxia leading to paratonic

---

*To elicit the Glabellar Tap sign the glabella (mid point between the orbital ridges) is tapped rhythmically with the finger. The normal person will blink synchronously with the tapping for a few moments and then stop blinking. The patient with Parkinsonism will either continue blinking synchronously or the eyelids will go into spasm.

rigidity and a shuffling gait (astasia abasia) and of exaggerated tendon reflexes.

*Paratonic rigidity (gegenhalten)* is a form of rigidity in which the patient seems unable to relax his muscles when the limbs are being held by another person. It is sometimes described as 'quasivolitional' because the impression that the examiner gets is that the patient is positively resisting his attempts to move the limbs passively. The rigidity is inconstant inasmuch that it does not occur in the same position of the limb every time and it in no way interferes with the range of active movement through which the patient can put the limb when it is not being held by someone else. It thus appears that this rigidity is an inability to relate to movements when in contact with another person and it is a form of apraxia.

A similar phenomenon may sometimes be observed by nurses when they roll such a patient on his side towards them and he immediately shows widespread muscular rigidity, often clinging on to the nurse's dress.

Another form of this apraxia is seen when someone tries to assist such a patient to rise and walk. He will seem to lean backwards and again go into a state of muscle spasm, whereas if he is asked to get up and walk without being in contact with another person he may do this without such great difficulty.

The typical gait of cerebral arteriosclerosis is described either as the *Petren* gait or as *astasia abasia*. Not only does the patient shuffle but from time to time his feet seem to become glued to the floor. It may appear as though a magnet under the floor is pulling his feet towards it. However, if he is asked to step over a stick held at a height of 12 inches or so, he can do it without difficulty.

The third element of this syndrome is extremely brisk tendon reflexes in the presence of flexor plantar responses.

These are the principal findings in the syndrome of cerebral arteriosclerosis but a number of reflexes may be elicitable in this condition which are generally indicative of widespread generalized cerebral impairment. These are: grasp reflex and forced groping; sucking reflex and the palmomental reflex. (The first three indicate particular involvement of the frontal cortex.)

*The grasp reflex.* A stimulus of moving touch, or touch and pressure, over the radial side of the hand (the movement being towards the fingers) leads to brief contraction of the flexor muscles of the hand and fingers. If the stimulus then moves to the flexing fingers, .pulling against them, there is a rapid increasing of strength of the contraction, so that the patient could be pulled bodily out of the bed or chair if it were continued. The reflex becomes more sensitive if repeated two or three times (temporal summation).

*Forced groping.* When the palm is touched (the patient with his eyes closed) the fingers close and the hand moves in the direction that the stimulus appears to come from.

*Sucking reflex.* An object (e.g. a pencil) in contact with the lips, produces the muscle contractions appropriate to sucking.

*Palmo-mental reflex.* A non-painful stimulus (a scratch) applied to the palm produces contraction of the mentalis muscle.

Other generalized accompaniments of this syndrome include perseveration, and urinary incontinence with an uninhibited neurogenic bladder.

## Syndromes predominantly within the carotid territory

There are three major disorders: transient ischaemic attacks, strokes and arteritis.

### Transient ischaemic attacks

A transient ischaemic attack (TIA) is an episode of focal loss of cerebral function lasting for minutes or hours from which full recovery occurs within 24 hours. While it may include loss of consciousness this is not common and the symptoms or signs are varied depending on the part of the brain affected. TIA's may occur either in the carotid territory or in the vertebro-basilar territory. Their aetiology is not entirely clear and may include several different mechanisms In the carotid territory they are particularly associated with atheromatous stenosis of the internal carotid artery and are believed to be due to microemboli arising from this plaque. Symptoms include monocular loss of vision, due to emboli in the retinal artery, speech disorder (dysarthria or dysphasia including transient word blindness); monoparesis or hemiparesis; paraesthesia or anaesthesia.

Symptoms are usually of the same type in each attack.

*Prognosis.* TIA's have great prognostic significance since one third to one half of patients with recurrent TIA's will develop a crippling stroke within three years. Those in the

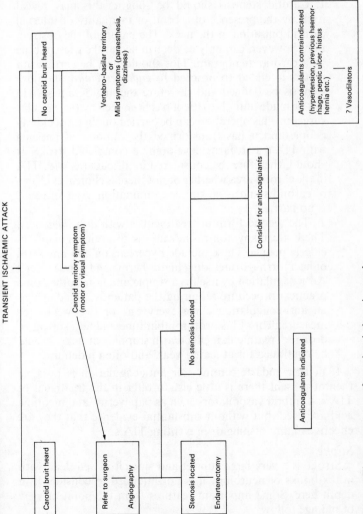

Fig. 4.6 The management of transient ischaemic attacks.

carotid area have a much more serious prognosis than those in the vertebro-basilar area.

*Treatment.* (see Figure 4.6) TIA's in the carotid territory should be treated as follows:

1. Carotid stenosis should be sought; this may reveal itself by the presence of a bruit or inequality of internal carotid pulsation in the neck. The nature of the obstruction, however, can only be determined at the present time by a carotid angiogram. This should only be carried out if it is intended to proceed to *endarterectomy* should a stenosis be defined and therefore the angiogram should not be made until the patient has been seen by the vascular surgeon. This operation can be carried out in most elderly people and it has transformed the outlook of patients with TIA's as regards developing a completed stroke. It should, therefore, be considered in all patients with TIA in the carotid area whether or not there is clinical evidence of carotid stenosis on simple examination. Age, of itself, is no barrier.

2. The second form of treatment is with *anticoagulants*. There are many contra-indications to anticoagulants in elderly people. These include hypertension and any form of haemorrhage (including hiatus hernia and peptic ulcer). Anticoagulation by itself is a simple and non-bothersome practical procedure requiring the patient's attendance at an anti-coagulation clinic every one or two weeks for measurement of his prothrombin time and adjustment of dosage. Treatment. if effective in stopping attacks, should be continued for at least a year, and often indefinitely.

If neither endarterectomy nor anticoagulation is possible then at present there is little else to offer in the treatment of TIA's. Cerebral vasodilators such as papaverine and nicotinic acid are used. but without substantial evidence that they are effective in diminishing or preventing TIA's.

*Stroke*

Stroke is a very large subject and since it is well dealt with in textbooks of neurology it is not intended to consider it in depth here. Some important features from the point of view of old age follow.

Stroke may be classified on a pathological basis, that is as an infarct due either to thrombosis or embolism, or as a haemorrhage, or it may be classified on a clinical basis as a 'stroke-in-evolution' or 'a completed stroke'. A *stroke-in-evolution* is one which develops over a number of hours or days. It may be associated with any of the three pathological causes since, although an embolism is sudden in its onset, there may be further thrombus formation proximal to the embolus, causing a gradual extension of the infarcted area; and while haemorrhage is also sudden in its onset there may be further seepage of blood and development of ischaemia over a period of time. Also in all cases of stroke, associated oedema will develop over a number of hours following the initial catastrophe and this may cause a progression of symptoms.

In the differential diagnosis of stroke it is important to exclude *subdural haematoma*, particularly in patients whose level of consciousness fluctuates over a number of days and who also demonstrate a hemiparesis. Subdural haematoma is often related to a history of trauma to the head but this is present quite often in patients with cerebral infarct or haemorrhage because they fall. The other important diagnostic differentiation is a *subarachnoid haemorrhage* which again may produce hemiparesis (occasionally in the old). There is usually intense generalized headache (which is also common in intracerebral haemorrhage). One important diagnostic feature is the presence of pupillary inequality.

In a subarachnoid haemorrhage the lumbar puncture will show evidence of bleeding or of xanthochromia if it is carried out after a few days. The blood or xanthochromia may or may not be present with an intracerebral haemorrhage. (The diagnosis of subarachnoid haemorrhage is important because of its surgical management).

Perhaps the most important aspects of stroke which are dealt with by the geriatrician are the management of the processes of rehabilitation and of speech disorder and these are dealt with in Chapter 21.

*Temporal arteritis*

Temporal (or giant cell) arteritis is a generalized disease of medium sized arteries which commonly affects branches of the external carotid artery. It is also occasionally a cause of stroke. Temporal arteritis is a condition of the second half of life and becomes commoner as people get older. It is a disease whose diagnosis must be made promptly, for if it is suspected the patient may, at any time, develop blindness or (much less commonly) a stroke and this can be prevented by treatment with steroids. Giant cell arteritis most commonly affects the temporal artery, which in the acute phase becomes tender, hot and thickened, but later is both painless and pulseless. The commonest presenting symptom is temporal headache. The disease may, however, affect any artery in the body and there is often constitutional disturbance: malaise, fatigue, generalized aches and pains. The retinal artery is the second most commonly affected and this may be bilateral leading to impairment or total loss of vision. The diagnosis of giant cell arteritis may be suspected by elevation of the ESR and confirmed by a biopsy of the affected artery. These investigations should not be awaited, however, before treatment is started. Blood should be removed for ESR and the patient started on 40 to 60 mg prednisolone a day. He can usually be weaned to a dose of 10 to 20 mg within a fortnight and should be maintained on a dose of 10 to 15 mg for the following year. Steroids may then be withdrawn but a recrudescence of activity must be looked for by frequent estimations of the ESR over the following 12 months.

Giant cell arteritis is thought to be a variant of another disease which is common in old people, *polymyalgia rheumatica*. This presents with widespread muscular pain and tenderness, sometimes with a fever but more generally with lassitude and non-specific symptoms. There are no focal arterial lesions as in temporal arteritis. Once again the ESR is raised and treatment with steroids causes almost immediate relief of symptoms and normalisation of the ESR. An arterial biopsy will show evidence of giant cell arteritis in some patients with polymyalgia rheumatica.

**Vertebro-basilar territory syndromes**

The vertebral and basilar arteries supply blood to the hind brain, the cerebellum and occipital cortices. Ischaemia in these areas may produce impairment of neuro-regulatory functions. These include particularly reflex posture, the maintenance of blood pressure and of temperature regulation and the vomiting centre. Vertebro-basilar artery insufficiency therefore may be associated with falling, ataxia, nystagmus, giddiness, nausea and vomiting, episodes of hypotension and impairment of thermoregulation. Involvement of both occipital cortices may produce cortical blindness (and of one, homonymous hemianopia with macular sparing) and involvement of the cranial nerve nuclei may produce dysphagia, dysarthria, ophthalmoplegia, facial hemiparesis, hemianaesthesia, perioral paraesthesia and vertigo.

The two most important syndromes in this area however are transient ischaemic attacks and drop attacks.

*TIA's*

The definition is the same as in relation to the carotid area but the transitory symptoms are different and include all those listed in the paragraph above.

The aetiology is not known and there has not been demonstrated any clear correlation with vascular stenosis as is the case in the carotid attacks. There is thus no surgical approach and the first line of treatment is by anticoagulants. The prognosis of TIA's in the vertebro-basilar system is not as grave as those involving the carotid and in particular stroke as a long term sequel is less important.

*Drop attacks*

A drop attack is a fall which occurs without warning, without loss of consciousness and once the patient is on the floor he usually is unable to get up again by his own efforts. This definition is occasionally slightly modified inasmuch as some patients may have momentary dizziness or vertigo before they fall and some are able to get themselves up, particularly if they are able to climb up heavy furniture with their hands. The patient who falls as a result of a drop attack very often crumples to the ground and does not come crashing down and consequently injuries are less common than might be expected. However, drop attacks account for about 22 per cent of fractures of the femur in old people.

It is thought that drop attacks are due to sudden occlusion of both vertebral arteries as a result of kinking and/or impingement of osteophytes; the proximate cause is movement of the neck. The sudden loss of blood to the hind brain/cerebellum complex leads to a sudden loss of the reflex mechanisms for the maintenance of posture and so the patient falls. It is suggested that he cannot get himself up again because reflex posture does not return until there is a sensory input into the proprioceptive system. This requires pressure on the soles of his feet and the transmission of weight through the lower limbs. Certainly, once a patient who has had a drop attack is assisted onto his feet he can usually continue to walk.

The treatment of drop attacks is two-fold: first to ensure that patients who fall will do themselves as little damage as possible —on no account should they go up and down stairs unaccompanied —in addition, fires should always be guarded and the environment made as safe as possible. The second thing is to provide the patient with a cervical collar which prevents neck movements. This should be reasonably close fitting and it is often best to provide a temporary collar in the first place since collars are not always well tolerated by old people. The collar does not need to be worn in bed of course but must be put on whenever the patient gets out of bed. It is probably not worth prescribing a collar for someone who has only one or two drop attacks a year, but if they are more than once a month or if they are increasing in frequency then a trial with a cervical collar is required.

Our knowledge of the causes and management of drop attacks is as yet unsatisfactory. Compression of vessels by neck movement is a good theory but it is almost impossible to reproduce a drop attack by getting a patient to move his neck in different directions.

*Cervical spondylosis*

Cervical spondylosis describes the condition of the cervical spine which follows multiple disc degeneration. It is often associated with the clinical syndrome of vertebro-basilar artery ischaemia. One of the clinical features described in cervical spondylosis is nystagmus and this may occasionally point to vertebro-basilar insufficiency.

## Parkinsonism

Parkinsonism is a common condition in old people. It is well described in neurological textbooks and it is not intended to give a full description here; however, there are some points that are worth emphasizing in relation to the elderly.

### Differential diagnosis

*Classical Parkinsonism* is the condition of paralysis agitans which commonly occurs in middle age but which may have its onset in old age. The fully developed picture is one of akinesia, tremor, rigidity and sialorrhoea with paucity of expression.

*Post encephalitic Parkinsonism.* This is now becoming increasingly rare but is still found in a small number of elderly people who have had it most of their lives. Post encephalitic Parkinsonism was a complication of encephalitis lethargica or sleepy sickness, of which there were several epidemics in the years following 1919. In addition to the classical signs of Parkinsonism there are a number of special features, e.g. oculogyric crises, sweating crises and marked skeletal deformities —scoliosis, wrist and hand deformities.

*Drug induced Parkinsonism.* This is common in old people, particularly due to phenothiazines and tricyclic antidepressants.

*Secondary Parkinsonism* occurs in a few syndromes such as the Shy-Drager syndrome.

*Arteriosclerotic Parkinsonism.* This has been referred to already (p. 38). It is an atypical clinical variant of Parkinsonism and is assumed to be associated with arterio-sclerotic involvement of the basal ganglia although so far no striking clinico-pathological association has been demonstrated.

### Treatment

The treatment of Parkinsonism is with L-dopa and its associated preparations. Effective treatment by L-dopa is limited mainly by nausea and vomiting. For this reason preparations containing L-dopa and a dopa-decarboxylase inhibitor are now widely used in geriatric practice. The dopa-decarboxylase inhibitor diminishes the peripheral breakdown of L-dopa to dopamine outside the CNS, and so allows a higher concentration of L-dopa (and so dopamine) within the central nervous system. Lower doses of L-dopa may thus be used which lead to fewer side-effects. The main side-effects of L-dopa are those arising within the central nervous system, particularly dyskinesia (i.e. bizarre movements).

L-Dopa and similar drugs can precipitate severe confusion, sometimes with hallucinations, and they should be used cautiously in any old person already mildly confused. Hiccups and haematuria are two other unwanted effects.

L-Dopa should not be used in conjunction with any psychotropic drugs which affect cerebral amine metabolism.

Anticholinergic anti-Parkinsonian drugs (benxhexol, orphenadrine, procyclidine etc.) have long been used in treating Parkinsonism but are not striking in their effect. Old people are very sensitive to benzhexol and it sometimes causes an acute confusional disturbance. Another important alternative is to use amantadine either alone or in combination with one of the above drugs.

It will be appreciated that arteriosclerotic Parkinsonism is a clinical rather than a pathological entity. Its effects are not susceptible to treatment with any of the above anti-Parkinsonian drugs.

FURTHER READING

Adams. G.F. (1974) *Cerebrovascular Disability and the Aging Brain.* Edinburgh: Churchill Livingstone.

# 5. Autonomic Disorders

Some degree of failure of the autonomic nervous system becomes increasingly more common as we get older. This is evident from a number of important clinical syndromes. Accidental hypothermia, postural hypotension, bladder dysfunction, difficulty in swallowing and disordered motility of the lower bowel are particularly important in old people. One question that immediately arises is to what extent are some of these changes the effect of aging itself or of various pathological processes? Also, to what extent are they multifactorial in their cause? Drugs and environmental factors may contribute, as well as the morphological and metabolic effects of aging. To most of these questions there is at present no answer, but it is important to have the question in mind when considering the various syndromes of autonomic failure in old age.

A rare form of autonomic failure in younger patients is the Shy-Drager Syndrome, whose symptoms include impotence, retention of urine, postural hypotension and faecal incontinence.

One or two general mechanisms have been demonstrated. For instance, it has been shown that with increasing age there is some alteration in neuro-transmission at autonomic ganglia with a decrease in the formation of acetylcholine, largely due to a decrease in the key enzyme choline acetylase but also due to diminution of the cholinesterase effect. These two changes tend to diminish autonomic function but against them must be set a third effect, namely that the cholino-receptive protein (of the post-synaptic membrane) seems to be more sensitive to acetylcholine as a result of aging. The overall result, therefore, will depend on both of these factors. In addition there appear to be morphological changes including a diminution in the overall number of cholino-receptors. The net result would seem to be diminution in the effectiveness of autonomic action with aging. However, as in so many other fields in the infant science of gerontology, there is much that has still to be discovered.

Among the pathological changes likely to affect autonomic function the most obvious is cerebrovascular disease. There is no doubt that a high proportion of patients suffering from hypothermia, postural hypotension and bladder disorders are also suffering from cerebrovascular disease. Many drugs, particularly phenothiazines and anti-Parkinsonian drugs, together with the whole range of anticholinergic preparations, can contribute to these changes.

The controlling centre of the autonomic nervous system is the hypothalamus and studies of changes in the hypothalamus with aging are still awaited.

## Orthostatic hypotension

Postural hypotension may be defined as a drop of 20 mm Hg in systolic or diastolic pressure on change from the recumbent to the erect posture. If a young person jumps out of bed rapidly he may experience momentary light-headedness due to postural hypotension for which the vasomotor regulating mechanism immediately compensates. In old age, however, this compensatory mechanism may be so inefficient that postural hypotension may last for an hour or more. Quite often it leads to a stuporose condition which is only reversed when the patient is lain horizontal once more. Postural hypotension is one of the causes of falls in the elderly, particularly in old people getting out of bed at night to go and empty their bladders.

Maintenance of blood pressure is a reflex mechanism. The afferent fibres begin in the baroreceptors of the carotid sinus and they pass through the glossopharyngeal nerve to the brain stem vasomotor centre. Efferent impulses pass through the spinal cord and the preganglionic fibres to the sympathetic chain, and through postganglionic fibres to the blood vessels where their action is one of vasoconstriction. Testing this reflex at various points has shown that in old people with postural hypotension the failure is central rather than peripheral, although there is some evidence that baroreceptor function is also affected by aging.

A survey carried out among 100 patients aged 70+ admitted to a geriatric ward showed a prevalence of postural hypotension of 17 per cent, but an even higher figure has been reported among old people at home. In nearly all patients with postural hypotension there is some evidence of cerebrovascular disease. A few show Parkinsonism and other associated diseases including diabetes and the effect of drugs.

Postural hypotension may produce light-headedness and dizziness, a condition of stupor, or it may cause the patient to fall. The diagnosis and management are described on pages 138 to 140.

### Impairment of thermoregulation

This may manifest itself in two ways, hypothermia or hyperthermia and the most commonly recognized of these is accidental hypothermia. A study carried out in London of over 1000 old people in the winter showed a deep body temperature of less than 35·5°C in 10 per cent of them. Low body temperatures were more common in the mornings, and were associated with cold bedrooms. They were also the poorest group in the survey in that a significant proportion were in receipt of supplementary benefit.

Many factors contribute to producing accidental hypothermia in the elderly. Blunted appreciation of cold is important. Others include environmental factors such as poor insulation in houses, inadequate clothing and inadequate heating, most of which are often associated with what is perhaps the commonest underlying cause, and that is poverty. A diminished metabolic rate, as in hypothyroidism and the effect of drugs, particularly chlorpromazine, are sometimes contributory factors. Immobility itself may also contribute and exposure is important, particularly among the elderly who may fall down in the night going to the lavatory and remain scantily clad on the floor of a freezing room for hours or, occasionally, days before someone finds them. In many of these circumstances hypothermia would occur in people at any age.

An additional factor in old age, however, is the effect of cerebrovascular disease and indeed of aging itself on the central mechanism of heat regulation.

The hypothalamus is thought to act rather like a thermostat:

it sets a temperature which various peripheral mechanisms then contribute towards maintaining (see Fig. 5.1). If the

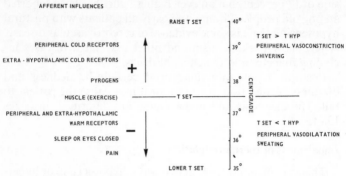

Fig. 5.1 Thermoregulation.

temperature is set high then the various mechanisms of pilo-erection, peripheral vasoconstriction, shivering and a feeling of cold, making the person put on more clothes, has the effect of bringing the body temperature up to the 'set' temperature. Similarly if the temperature is set low, mechanisms such as vasodilatation, sweating and shedding of clothing help to bring the body temperature down to this lower level. The 'set' of the temperature may be raised by pyrogens or by the sensory mechanisms of the body recording a low environmental temperature. The 'set' of the temperature may be lowered if the body becomes heated as a result of exercise or of a hot environment, which is again recorded through the sensory side of the thermoregulatory reflexes. The centre for thermoregulation is in the hypothalamus and it is probably in this area that impairment due to cerebrovascular disease of aging occurs. The presence of these defects has been demonstrated in a study from Oxford where a group of patients who had survived hypothermia and who were alert and active, were compared to a group of normal old people acting as controls, in a number of tests involving body cooling. The fact that thermoregulatory mechanisms were impaired in the hypothermia survivors is demonstrated in Figure 5.2 which shows a drop in deep body temperature on cooling (not occurring in the control group). Figure 5.3 compares this with changes in skin temperature as a

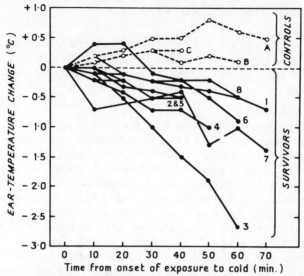

Fig. 5.2 Effect of cooling on deep body temperature. (After MacMillan *et al.*, 1967.)

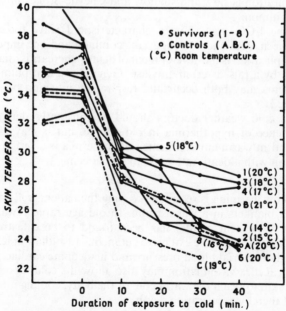

Fig. 5.3 Effect of cooling on skin temperature. (After MacMillan *et al.*, 1967.)

result of cooling in both groups (no difference). In addition the survivors showed no shivering, little reduction in hand blood flow and no significant change in oxygen consumption during cooling—all evidence of thermoregulatory failure.

*Clinical features*

Accidental hypothermia is a condition in which the deep body temperature falls to 35°C or below. It can usually be diagnosed by feeling the patient's body but it can only be established by using a low-reading thermometer. A special low-reading clinical thermometer is available: alternatively the rectal temperature may be taken using a lotion thermometer. Hypothermic patients are pale and show a somatic tremor but shivering is absent. Consciousness may be impaired or the patient may simply be apathetic, possibly displaying disorientation, hallucination or paranoid features. Muscle rigidity, diminished reflexes, slurred speech and occasionally extensor plantar responses are found. There is bradycardia, respiration is slow and shallow and Cheyne-Stokes breathing is common.

The ECG may show a characteristic J wave (occurring between QRS and T); oliguria is common and one important complication is the development of acute pancreatitis, diagnosable by a raised serum amylase. Generalized and pulmonary oedema may both occur and respiratory infection be superadded.

In cold weather doctors should be constantly alert to the presence of hypothermia in old people, but it may also be found in warm environments. Hypothermia is a serious condition with a death rate of 35 to 40 per cent.

*Management*

Slow warming is required, keeping the patient well covered with blankets in a warm room. In old age rapid rewarming (e.g. by a heat cradle) has been found to be catastrophic, possibly because the extensive cutaneous vasodilation leads to a fall of arterial blood pressure and inadequate cardiac perfusion. Reflex vasodilation may also allow the cold blood from the skin to reach the warm core of the body, cooling it further and thereby accelerating death.

Cardiac monitoring is helpful to identify the frequent occurrence of cardiac dysrhythmia, treatment of which can occasionally be life saving.

Care must be taken that the patient does not aspirate vomit. A clear airway must be maintained and an antibiotic give to prevent the development of bronchopneumonia. Intravenous fluids must be used with great caution. Hypokalaemia must be looked for while treatment proceeds. Intravenous hydrocortisone (200 mg) is usually given within the first 48 hours to patients suffering from moderate and severe hypothermia and followed by 15 mg prednisolone a day for the next two days.

Hypothyroidism, if suspected, must of course be treated but treatment must not start until the temperature has risen to at least 32·2°C. Tri-iodothyronine in small doses is then usually given parenterally.

*Prevention*. Accidental hypothermia in old people is a much larger problem in very cold weather than is generally realized and in promoting positive health doctors should be concerned about the environment in which their aged patients live. Extra money is available from Social Security Departments as fuel allowance for the poor and Social Services Departments are empowered to assist with installation of heaters and of insulation where this is needed. Adequate and suitable clothing is also required. An electric blanket used with care is helpful, and special low voltage electric blankets are now available at low cost.

Always carry a low-reading thermometer.

Autonomic effects as seen in the oesophagus, bladder and lower bowel are dealt with in the relevant chapters of this book.

FURTHER READING

Brocklehurst, J.C. (1975) Aging of the Autonomic Nervous System. *Age and Aging*. Suppl. pp. 7–17.
Johnson *et al.* (1965) Effect of posture on blood-pressure in elderly patients. *Lancet*, i. pp. 731–3.
MacMillan *et al.* (1967) Temperature regulation in survivors of accidental hypothermia of the elderly. *Lancet*, i. pp. 165–9.

# 6. Falls

Falls are one of the important presenting symptoms of disease in the elderly. The student should therefore be fully conversant with the differential diagnosis of falls in old people. There are one or two general points to be made first of all.

*Sway*

Maintenance of the erect posture requires the balancing of a very large mass with a high centre of gravity over a very small base. This fine balance is maintained by the anti-gravity muscles and by sensory input from the skin, muscles and joints. These inform as soon as the centre of gravity begins to move away from the base and the appropriate muscles then contract to correct this movement. Of course vision and vesti-bular function also contribute. The whole complex process is learned in childhood and becomes reflex and unconscious throughout most of life. It is centred in the cerebellum and hind brain.

As with so many other automatic body functions the reflex maintenance of posture becomes impaired as people move into old age. They are less able to correct quickly, and adequately, movements of their centre of gravity away from the base and this may be one of the reasons why old people fall. This may be seen particularly as an increase in sway.

Many years ago Sheldon investigated the prevalence of sway in groups of people of different ages and his findings (shown in Fig. 6.1) form a graphic illustration of the way in which maintenance of the erect posture is acquired during childhood and becomes slightly impaired in old age.

*Muscle weakness*

Locking of the knee joints, the last movement in a series of strong muscle actions in the powerful antigravity muscles of the lower limbs, also contributes to standing erect. While there

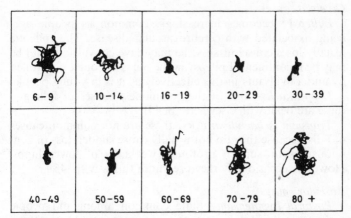

Fig. 6.1 Sway—effects of age.

is little evidence that loss of muscle power associated with aging is *per se* the cause of falls it is likely that this is one of a number of predisposing factors in some old people. Others may include weakness due to osteomalacia or peripheral neuropathy and (much more commonly) the effects of osteoarthrosis of the knee and hips.

All of these things may, therefore, be predisposing factors to falling in the elderly. The differential diagnosis of falls will, therefore, include other factors which may be precipitating factors, as well as conditions which are the entire cause of falls.

## Differential diagnosis of falls

### Environmental causes

These include inadequate lighting, inconvenient objects such as mats, carpets and others left lying around: it may also include pavements and unevenness of the road and garden. Falls associated with these environmental hazards are usually called trips.

### Inadequate vision

People who are old and blind lose their balance easily. It might be thought also that they would trip more often than sighted people but in fact they seem to be more careful in their movements and there is evidence to suggest that they do not trip as often as sighted people.

## Cerebral causes

*Epilepsy:* becomes increasingly common as people age, being associated with cerebrovascular disease. The epileptic usually loses consciousness: he may have convulsions and he may be incontinent. Epilepsy in the old is of course controlled by anticonvulsants just as effectively as it is in young people.

*Drop-attacks*—one of the commonest causes of falling— these are dealt with elsewhere (p. 45).

*Transient ischaemic attacks:* these are not common causes of falls because they do not usually cause sudden loss of consciousness or sudden profound weakness of lower limbs. However, occasionally they present in this way (p. 45).

## Vascular causes

*Postural hypotension*—quite common among old people and of course also important in any patient who is taking hypotensive drugs. History of falling after assuming the upright posture (particularly getting out of bed) will raise suspicion. The blood pressure should be measured after the patient has lain down for 10 minutes or longer and then after standing for 2 minutes. The effect of postural hypotension may last for an hour or more, so this may be a cause of falls occurring quite a long time after the patient has got out of bed (p. 50).

*Syncope.* The ordinary faint occurs in the elderly just as in younger people.

*Micturition syncope.* Occasionally the rapid emptying of a distended bladder causes a drop in blood pressure and syncope. This is more likely to be the case at night if there is also an element of postural hypotension.

*Stokes-Adams attack.* Consciousness is lost, the patient is pulseless during the attack and when examined after it will be found to suffer from complete heart block. These attacks are due to asystole. Occasionally the ventricles do not start beating again and the patient dies. These attacks should be prevented by appropriate treatment of complete heart block but sometimes they are the first indication of that condition and they may be a cause of sudden death.

Occasionally a fall is the first indication of a major catastrophe, such as a myocardial or cerebral infarction, and may be the only presenting symptom.

# 7. Mental Confusion

Mental confusion is the very stuff of geriatric medicine. Four features make it bulk so large: its great prevalence (it accounts for just under half of all admissions to geriatric wards): the large variety of diseases which can provoke it: its socially disabling effects when long continued, and the very large demands it makes on medical and social resources.

What *is* 'mental confusion'? First and foremost, it is a disorder of cerebral function and not a diagnosis: the phrase does not define a disease entity. The human brain is a staggeringly complex 'information machine' capable of registering, storing and recalling billions of news items and of making an appropriate choice of action in response to them. Its operation is too intricate to be described in even the most elaborate computer jargon and the physiological bases of such familiar concepts as 'consciousness', 'memory' and 'attention' are only crudely understood. Small wonder that so marvellous a machine is readily vulnerable to minor changes in the supply of various fuels or the number of its basic functioning units, the neurones, or that when 'brain failure' occurs it is consistently ushered in by loss of the most sophisticated function of the brain, i.e. the ability to orient its owner in time and situation in relation to the external world and to dictate a course of action appropriate to the social framework in response to stimuli from the outside. When this topmost function is disrupted, there is 'confusion'

It has already been emphasized that many diseases can cause mental confusion and Table 7.1 gives a list, comprehensive but by no means exhaustive, of the causes. Broadly, there are two groups of confused patients:

> The *chronic brain syndrome*, also called 'chronic brain failure' and synonymous with dementia. This is a long drawn out disease with an inevitable downhill course and disastrous social consequences.

59

Table 7.1  Common causes of mental confusion

| | |
|---|---|
| 1. *The chronic brain syndrome* | |
| 2. *'Symptomatic' confusional states* | |
| Infections | Especially pneumonia and pyelocystitis, but many bacterial, parasitic and viral infections also |
| Cerebral hypoxia | Cardiac failure |
| | Severe anaemia |
| | Respiratory failure |
| Carcinomatosis | |
| Cerebral ischaemia | Stroke, embolism, diffuse cerebrovascular disease |
| Primarily metabolic | Hypokalaemia, hypoglycaemia, uraemia, diabetic precoma, water depletion, water intoxication |
| | Myxoedema |
| Nutritional (vitamin deficiency) | Pellagra (nicotinic acid deficiency) |
| | Scurvy (vitamin C lack) |
| | Vitamin $B_{12}$ and folic acid deficiency (role uncertain) |
| Environmental and social | Social upheaval or disaster |
| | Bereavement |
| | Abrupt change of environment |
| Depression | Pseudo-demented depression |
| Iatrogenic | Barbiturates, digitalis, L-dopa and many others |
| Organic cerebral lesion | Parkinson's disease |
| | Tumour, primary or secondary |
| | Subdural haematoma |

The *symptomatic confusional states* are temporary disruptions of cerebral function caused by more general diseases. In many instances complete recovery is possible if the underlying disease is recognized and treated. Ignorance of the cellular or biochemical causes of these confusional states is cloaked by the word 'toxic'.

A quiet note of caution needs to be sounded that, although it is useful for practical diagnostic purposes, to think of confusion in these two sharply defined groups, there are 'seed and soil' arguments for believing that symptomatic confusional states will be more easily precipitated in old people who are already verging on intellectual inadequacy. An infection, a social upset, or other factor may simply be the last straw that breaks the camel's back.

*Physiopathology*

A recurrent theme in this book is the difficulty of distinguishing 'aging' from 'disease', and the mental changes in old age epitomise this problem. Structural alterations in the brain consistently occur and are progressive from maturity to old age. The brain weight falls; there is, in some areas at any rate, a large fall-out of cortical neurones, and there is a steady accretion of two microscopic lesions, *'plaques'*, which are lamellated deposits of an amyloid substance, and *'neurofibrillary tangles'*. Neither the origin nor the functional significance of these lesions is clear. Within the neuronal cells a brown pigment 'lipofuscin' accumulates; this is probably no more than the product of degenerated lysosomes, but it has been implicated as a 'cause' of senile confusion.

Along with these 'normal' changes in the aging brain there are losses of mental capacity, though whether the structural lesions actually cause the functional loss or are merely associated, is not known.

'Intelligence' declines steadily throughout adult life, though different kinds of ability are lost at different rates. Verbal ability goes relatively slowly, while true conceptual and reasoning ability declines faster. Old people can compensate to some extent for loss of intellectual capacity by drawing on past experience, but when tests are 'paced' or done under distracting circumstances their performance fails.

Is 'dementia' simply an accentuated form of these normal changes or is it a 'disease'? The question is still open.

The role of cerebral arteriosclerosis as a cause of dementia is also debatable, though two kinds of dementia are often separated: 'senile' and 'arteriosclerotic'. Their distinction depends on the presence of collateral evidence of other arterial disease and an allegedly stepwise, downhill course in arteriosclerotic dementia, but the distinction is tenuous and serves little useful practical purpose.

*The pattern of causation*

The relative prevalence of the causes listed in Table 7.1 will depend on who assembles them—family doctor, psychiatrist and geriatrician will gather different patterns. Where admissions to geriatric wards are concerned, a recent multicentre survey showed that mental confusion accounted for 45 per cent of unselected acute admissions. The mentally impaired group were made up as follows:

Chronic brain failure      257
Symptomatic confusion  144

i.e. the chronic brain syndrome was nearly twice as common as all the 'symptomatic' confusional states lumped together.

Within the group of 'symptomatic' confusion, the major causes (not exclusive of each other) were: pneumonia (26 per cent); heart failure (33 per cent); urinary infection (25 per cent); carcinomatosis (12 per cent); depression (12 per cent).

*A step-by-step approach to the diagnosis of confusion*

The following sequence is suggested:
1. A detailed history of the complaint, with special reference to:
   rate of evolution of the mental disturbance
   evidence of failing intellectual or social capacity
   drug therapy
   major social upheavals
   co-existence of physical symptoms
   previous admissions to hospital and reasons
   known history of previous mental disorder
   the patient's previous personality
   mood changes
2. Physical examination and observation of behaviour
3. Ancillary investigations for detection of occult physical disease
4. Use of psychometric tests.

*The history is all important*, and is best taken from someone who knows the patient well. By the very nature of the illness, the patient's own account is likely to be inaccurate and played-down.

The onset of the illness will often be polarized into two patterns:

The abrupt onset of confusion in a patient previously vigorous, mentally clear and socially independent: this suggests a symptomatic confusional state and urgently demands exclusion of an organic lesion. At the other pole is the protracted development of 'odd' or 'funny' behaviour, in lay language, suggesting a dementing process. This long course can, however, eventually erupt as a social crisis and then masquerade as an acute confusion. The gradually developing mental changes can be quite subtle: minor offences against the social code, a barely perceptible fall in the standard of dress or personal hygiene, a coarsening of language or inability to handle money affairs as astutely as before. An articulate lay person well acquainted with the patient will often help to distinguish between mere personal eccentricity and what is truly abnormal for the person in question. Grosser evidence will often be forthcoming in the shape of aimless wandering and getting lost; progressive incompetence in self-care, hoarding, proneness to domestic accidents, and inability to use kitchen instruments safely.

### Drug therapy

Since a host of drugs can cause confusion it is important to know not only about those currently prescribed, but about any lapsed prescriptions held in reserve at the patient's discretion, and any 'over-the-counter' drugs. Barbiturates, 'sleeping tablets' of any kind, digitalis and anti-Parkinsonism drugs are common offenders.

Alcoholism is by no means rare in old people, who can be as adept at concealing their addiction as the young.

### Social upheavals and disasters

Under this heading one includes bereavement (a spouse, friends, children, pets), dismissal from employment, financial worries, retirement difficulties and removal to an unfamiliar neighbourhood.

The final three points on the history check-list are concerned with detection of 'pseudo-demented depression'.

This is of special importance since it is a treatable and often reversible condition with a good prognosis if it be recognized. But it is easily mislabelled as dementia, because apathy and failure of attention can give a falsely poor performance on tests of intellectual ability or memory.

A direct question will be needed to get information about previous treatment for mental disorder. Direct questions such as 'are you feeling depressed?' rarely get much response from old people: 'how are your spirits?' or 'are you pleased with life?' are more rewarding.

*Physical examination*

A glance at Table 7.1 will show that the causal conditions within the group of 'symptomatic confusion' cover almost the whole of internal medicine: a catalogue of the main physical signs of each cause would be soporific and serve little purpose, so apart from an exhortation to omit nothing (the bony skull, visual fields, retinae, ears and pelvis are the usual sins of omission), only a few points need be made:

> Pneumonia is a common cause of confusion, but in the elderly the respiratory signs—fever, sputum and signs of pulmonary consolidation—are often minor or atypical and reliance on their presence may be misleading.
>
> In patients whose history is compatible with a chronic brain syndrome, there often remains a nagging doubt that there could be an underlying structural cerebral lesion, such as tumour, abscess or subdural haematoma. Suspicion of these is legitimately raised by: severe headaches, failing vision, epileptiform attacks or a history of trauma.

Some more general features help to distinguish dementia from other kinds of confusion: in the demented patient the use of language is poor, only simple ideas are vocalized, neologisms are common and replies to questions are often tangential. Patients will often ask for a question to be repeated in order to gain time to reply, or will answer one question by asking another.

In symptomatic confusion on the other hand, as in an otherwise healthy person with pneumonia, there is often normal or unusually vivid use of language and its thought content is rich.

Incontinence of urine or faeces is more likely to occur in dementia than in other confusional states. Two other features of general behaviour often present in dementia are nocturnal wandering and 'restless fiddling'.

*Ancillary investigations* are mainly of use in detecting the lesions underlying symptomatic confusion. Each patient requires individual thought, but the most rewarding drag-net of routine investigations will be a chest X-ray, a blood count and a urine culture.

*Use of psychometric tests*

A number of simple, quickly performed tests of question-naire type are now widely used, e.g. the Royal College of Physicians' 'Mental Status Questionnaire'. Most contain questions designed to measure orientation, recent memory retention and conceptual ability. The tests are easily performed and give a numerical result. While they are useful as a screening procedure and for following progress when skilfully used, such tests do not discriminate the demented from the non-demented with the same accuracy as a 'global' assessment by an experienced clinician, and there is the risk of being 'dazzled by decimal points' and attaching undue importance to the numerical result. Certainly, no patient should ever be labelled 'demented' from the results of these tests alone.

## The management of confusion

The need to distinguish symptomatic confusional states from the chronic brain syndrome has already been emphasized: this is the first and most important step in management. Assuming that this has been thoroughly done, management has two other elements:

1. The control of disordered behaviour
2. Management of the whole patient in a social environment.

*Disordered behaviour:* its control by drugs

Confusional states are no exception to the principle that old people are better off without drugs, if their use can possibly be avoided and many mild confusional states, especially 'simple forgetfulness', will not need any psychotropic drug therapy. The main question—which drug?—is difficult to answer because of the large range of similar drugs available. Before making detailed suggestions (which will inevitably reveal a personal preference) some general dos and don'ts are:

*Do:*  Gain experience in the handling of a few established drugs rather than flirt with every newcomer

*Do:*  Give the drug in full dosage, but make a rough allowance for body weight

*Do:*  Taper off injection therapy, don't stop suddenly or the patient may tack from one extreme to the other.

*Don't:*  Give potent psychotropic drugs in untried cocktail combinations: interactions are frequent and difficult to predict.

*Don't:*  Give barbiturates to confused old people: these drugs are addictive, they cause microsomal induction and so upset the dosage of other drugs. They are themselves a cause of confusion.

*Don't:*  Give intramuscular paraldehyde to old people: it is an unpleasant and obsolete remedy.

*The circumstances in which drug therapy is useful*

*Nocturnal wandering and restlessness.* This is probably the commonest cause of final rejection of a confused old person living with relatives. Noctambulism frightens and creates havoc from continued sleeplessness. The most useful drugs for its control are either: *chlormethiazole* in syrup form, in a dosage of 500–1000 mg about one hour before retiring. Many old people will want to go to bed unusually early: not always a good habit since their sleep requirements are in any case usually small. For the same reason, medication during the day should not produce actual sleep.

An alternative is *promazine* given in a dose of 50 mg and increasing each day by 25 mg (up to 100 mg) until the effective dose is found. If this drug is ineffective by itself, it may be combined with chlormethiazole in the dose mentioned.

*Daytime restlessness, agitation and hyperactivity.* Two useful drugs for these disturbances are *haloperidol* and *thioridazine*. Haloperidol can be given as capsules of 0·5 mg two or three times daily, or, more effectively, the required dose can be titrated using a syrup, containing about 0·2 mg per drop, starting with a dose of 0·4 mg t.d.s. until behaviour is controlled.

Thioridazine is given orally in a dose of 25–50 mg thrice daily.

*Frankly aggressive behaviour and/or uncontrollable restlessness with hallucinations (the 'florid delirious state').* This is a relatively rare event in confused old people, but requires effective control, and usually needs intramuscular therapy. Three proven drugs are: chlorpromazine, dose 50 to 100 mg i.m.i.; haloperidol, 2·5 to 5 mg i.m.i. or diazepam, 5 to 10 mg i.m.i.

The first two cause Parkinsonism and postural hypotension, and chlorpromazine causes cholestatic jaundice. It is sometimes recommended to give an anticholinergic drug together with chlorpromazine or haloperidol, to combat the extrapyramidal side effects, but the giving of an active drug to combat the side effects of primary therapy is a slippery slope to venture on.

Some old people develop morbid ideas of persecution or personal ill-treatment while they are confused: they may have been paranoid for long before or the suspiciousness can be simply a reaction to an unfamiliar and therefore hostile environment. Mild paranoid symptoms can be helped by thioridazine (see above) and more severe states by trifluoperazine in a dose of 1 to 3 mg two or three times daily. If the confusion is part of a pseudo-demented depression, tricyclic antidepressant drugs or electroconvulsive therapy may be needed, and treatment is best carried out by a psychiatrist.

*Management of the whole patient*

The chronic brain syndrome threatens or destroys the patients' ability to organize their lives effectively for independent survival, and their management often involves placement in a suitably protected environment. It is worth remembering that insight is usually lost early in the chronic brain syndrome: the patients consequently suffer little, but the relatives responsible for their care may suffer greatly from the restrictions and tensions introduced into their lives.

There are two central questions: 'is the patient fit to live alone, and if so what social support will be needed?' and 'if not fit to live alone where should he be?' The answers to these questions depend largely on the degree of dementia and Table 7.2 gives a guide to the assessment of its severity and the possible social solutions. But it has to be admitted that the reasonable demand for institutional care far outstrips the supply. Many demented old people must perforce live 'in the community' but their existence is precarious in the extreme and they lurch from one crisis to another, until social pressures compel their admission to an institution of some kind.

Two other syndromes requiring brief mention in this chapter are paraphrenia and the Diogenes syndrome.

Table 7.2 Degrees of dementia and possible social solutions

| Degree of dementia | Features | Social possibilities |
| --- | --- | --- |
| Mild | Distrait and forgetful. Tends to neglect housework but can still manage primitive cooking safely. Continent, personal hygiene adequate. Aware of personal identity and own address, and can find way about neighbourhood. Conversation limited but relevant. Can make special effort for special occasions. | Can survive at home if competent, devoted spouse or relative. If widowed or single will need help: neighbours, Home Help, meals on wheels. Support in Day Hospital or Day Centre. |
| Moderate (no physical disability) | 'Happy wandering'—gets lost outside home, does not know own address. Accident-prone: leaves gas taps on, boils kettle dry, careless with fires. Kitchen neglected. Does not buy food. Sleeps in day clothes. Often incontinent of urine. | If single or widowed, not safe to live alone but may struggle on with devoted relative or spouse. If alone will need place in Old People's Home, Home for Elderly Mentally Infirm, or private nursing home if large funds available. |
| Moderate (with physical disability such as falls, stroke, severe arthritis) | As above but mobility limited and may be chair- or bed-fast | Not fit to live alone. If with relative will need great support, possibly frequent hospital admissions. Not suitable for residential home. Probably needs long-stay bed ultimately. |
| Severe (no physical disability) | Gross memory defect. Total neglect of hygiene. Often doubly incontinent. Makes no effort to cook or care for self. Conversation rambling, incoherent. | Exceptional relative may cope at personal expense. Patient will need long-stay bed, probably in psychiatric unit. |
| Severe (with physical disability) | As above, but chairfast or bedfast. | Requires long-stay bed under care of geriatrician |

*Paraphrenia* or late onset schizophrenia is a form of persecutory state in which the patient has paranoid delusions usually about a neighbour. The delusions are commonly of some fear of attack such as by 'passing electricity under the floor'. The condition usually occurs in people who have always led withdrawn and isolated lives—often spinsters. The delusions occasionally lead to noisy abuse of the neighbours, or the spreading of scandal. The condition is often simply treated with phenothiazines.

The *Diogenes syndrome* is one in which the external appearances are of grossly disordered behaviour—living in a house which has become filthy, often with many cats, a large accumulation of newspapers and other rubbish. Old people suffering from this condition have a high IQ and in about 50 per cent of cases are otherwise intellectually normal. They do not want to come into hospital (though sometimes they have concomitant physical disease needing treatment). If they are admitted while their home is cleaned up, in a few months it will revert again to its previous chaos. Unless they are a danger to other people they should not be forced into an institution. Medical care often has to be adapted to treatment at home.

# 8. Urinary Incontinence

Urinary incontinence is one of the most important presenting symptoms of illness in the elderly. As with other members of the geriatric triad (falls and mental confusion) it is important to stress that it is a *symptom* and requires careful investigation in order to diagnose its cause. It is also an extremely disabling condition, unpleasant for the sufferer and for those with whom she has to live. It may be the one single factor which makes it necessary for an old person to live in a long stay hospital ward rather than at home or in a residential home. Incontinence of urine, therefore, is a most important symptom in the elderly. There is an enormous potential for treatment by the doctor who is fully aware of its possible causes and is prepared to investigate and to treat it thoroughly.

*Dysuric symptoms.* Incontinence of urine is one of a number of symptoms relating to the control of micturition which may be disordered in old age. Others include nocturnal frequency of micturition, daytime frequency and urgency of micturition. In many cases these may lead on, in the course of time to incontinence.

*Prevalence.* A large number of surveys (summarized in Table 8.1) have indicated the prevalence of these various

Table 8.1 Symptoms of dysuria in a series of 557 people aged 65+ (182 male, 375 female). All figures are percentages.

|  | Male | Female | Total |
|---|---|---|---|
| Nocturia | 70 | 61 | 64 |
| Precipitancy | 28 | 32 | 30 |
| Urgency | 14 | 9 | 10 |
| Difficulty | 13 | 3 | 7 |
| Scalding | 7 | 13 | 11 |
| Total incontinence | 17 | 23 | 20 |
| Stress incontinence | 3 | 12 | 9 |

symptoms of dysuria. They are more common among patients in hospital than those at home, for reasons which will become apparent. Further, these figures may reflect suboptimal treatment in the past and the situation in more recent years may well be improving.

All of these symptoms are more common in the older age group (80+).

## Causes of incontinence

It is convenient to consider the causes of incontinence on an anatomical basis, in four main sub-divisions as follows:
1. Disorders of the pelvic diaphragm
2. Disorders of the urethra and bladder outlet
3. Disorders within the bladder itself
4. Disorders of the neurological control of micturition.

### Disorders of the pelvic diaphragm

In both sexes the bladder lies on the pelvic diaphragm (the pubococcygeus and levator ani muscles). The bladder outlet is normally maintained with the urethra at a right angle to the bladder base by the tone of these muscles and the elasticity of the connective tissues surrounding the urethra. This angle is important in maintaining closure of the bladder outlet. The base plate muscle of the bladder (part of the detrusor muscle, see Fig. 8.1) tends to maintain the internal urethral meatus

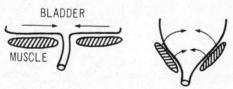

Fig. 8.1 The base plate of the bladder.

closed as long as the base plate is flat, but as soon as the right angle of the bladder outlet is lost, the base plate muscle loses its effect in maintaining closure of the internal urethral meatus; instead it contributes towards the contracting bladder. In normal micturition this process is initiated by contraction of the trigone muscle, which pulls open the internal urethral meatus and dislocates the base plate (see Fig. 8.1).

When the pelvic diaphragm muscles are weak, as is the case in women with any degree of uterine prolapse, then some degree of cystocele is apparent and the patient may suffer from stress incontinence. Stress incontinence may also occur in women who do not show the presence of cystocele and it may be that in such women incompetence of the bladder outlet is associated with changes in the elastic fibres, which help to maintain urethral closure. The external urethral sphincter is not an important muscle in the maintenance of continence (although it is useful in stopping micturition in mid-stream). Nor is there a separate anatomical internal urethral sphincter (although some muscle fibres from the detrusor muscle of the bladder continue into the urethra and have something of a sphincteric effect). Closure of the bladder outlet is very much a result of the firm supporting tissues around the urethra, together with the closing effect of the base plate and the tone of the pelvic diaphragm.

In incompetence of the pelvic diaphragm, or of the tissues surrounding the urethra, there is funnelling of the bladder outlet and this leads to effective shortening of the female urethra (see Fig. 8.2). In this condition any sudden rise in

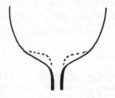

Fig. 8.2 Funnelling of bladder outlet and shortening of urethra.

intravesical pressure will cause immediate leakage of urine, i.e. stress incontinence.

*Stress incontinence* is an important disability in women of all ages, and indeed two surveys carried out among college students and student nurses have shown that 15 per cent of them had some degree of stress incontinence at least once a week and 50 per cent had it from time to time.

The diagnosis of stress incontinence is made on the history

and on examination of the vulva, when a degree of cystocele and urethrocele may be obvious. Leakage when the patient coughs may also be seen. However, these clinical findings are not always present and if the history is suggestive then a *urethral profile* will show a short and low-resistance urethra and a *micturating cystogram* (i.e. filling the bladder with a radioopaque fluid and taking X-rays while the patient actually micturates) may be necessary to indicate small degrees of incompetence of the internal urethral meatus.

The *unstable bladder* (see p. 83) is sometimes a cause of diagnostic confusion, since in the unstable bladder a cough or movement such as a change in posture may cause an uninhibited bladder contraction to be fired off, with almost immediate bladder emptying. The important difference is that in stress incontinence only a small amount of urine leaks out, (while intravesical pressure is raised) whereas in the unstable bladder a cough or movement fires off a bladder contraction leading to total emptying.

In the first place, treatment of stress incontinence involves referral to the physiotherapist. She will teach the patient pelvic floor exercises (similar to antenatal exercises with conscious contraction of the muscles of the pelvic diaphragm, including conscious cessation of micturition in mid-stream). This may be augmented by one of a variety of forms of electronic stimulation. The traditional form of this stimulation is by Faradism, which produces a surge of current along with which the patient learns to contract her muscles.

A similar effect may be obtained by using a pessary which is worn either vaginally or intra-anally and which contains ring electrodes wired to a battery worn externally. This is called a 'Continentor' and is worn for an hour or two each day, during which time the patient practises her exercises.

This combined treatment is often very successful and it is only when it fails that recourse to an internally worn pessary or to gynaecological surgery should be considered.

### Disorders of the urethra and bladder outlet

The sexes must be considered separately. In the female the most important condition is senile vaginitis. The lining of the adult female urethra is stratified squamous epithalium.

as is that of the vagina and as they are, so it is oestrogen sensitive (the bladder epithelium is transitional epithelium and is not oestrogen sensitive). As women grow older, stratified squamous epithelium extends in many of them on to the trigone.

Being oestrogen sensitive the epithelium becomes cornified during the menstrual cycle and in times of oestrogen deprivation it becomes atrophic. This is the condition seen in senile vaginitis and similar changes may affect the urethra and indeed the trigone. These in turn cause frequency and urgency of micturition and sometimes incontinence. The diagnosis is made by inspection of the vulva (and can be confirmed by a Papanicolou smear, though this is usually unnecessary).

*Treatment* is by courses of oestrogens or by the use of oestrogen cream locally. Oestrogens by mouth are preferable, since local application may introduce secondary infection in old women in whom perineal hygiene is a problem. The recommended drug is dienoestrol 0·3 mg t.d.s. and this should be given daily for a month, the course being repeated twice yearly.

In the male the main lesion in this group is enlargement of the prostate. *Benign prostatic hypertrophy* may cause bladder outlet obstruction leading to *chronic retention with overflow incontinence*. On the other hand, it may distort the bladder outlet so that the internal urethral meatus is no longer competent and urinary incontinence occurs with a low capacity bladder. The symptoms of frequency and urgency are also accompaniments of prostatic hypertrophy. Malignant disease of the prostate may cause similar symptoms.

Prostatic enlargement requires surgical removal of the gland and it is rare for a man who requires prostatectomy to be unfit for the operation, which may be performed urethrally with minimal postoperative upset. However, not infrequently there is more than one pathology affecting the control of micturition, and so some men who have incontinence together with a hypertrophied prostate may have also neurogenic changes impairing micturition (see below). If this is the case then prostatectomy, while it is necessary to relieve the bladder outlet obstruction, will not necessarily lead to a cure of these symptoms (if they are indeed neurogenic).

A common cause of urinary incontinence in both sexes is *impaction of faeces* (see p. 90). The impacting pelvic mass may either cause incontinence with a low capacity bladder or chronic retention with overflow incontinence. When the faecal impaction is treated the urinary (and usually faecal) incontinence will disappear.

### Disorders of the bladder itself

Almost any intrinsic disorder of the bladder may reveal itself as incontinence or as symptoms of urgency, nocturnal and daytime frequency. These include particularly *carcinoma* and the presence of a *calculus*: these two possibilities must always be considered. The diagnosis requires cystoscopy but this is a straightforward procedure, particularly in females, where it is easily done in an out-patient department.

Another and much more common disorder of the bladder which may cause these symptoms is *cystitis*. The implications of urinary infection are dealt with in detail on p. 191, where it is shown that there may either be an *acute infection* which is likely to be associated with symptoms including systemic effects (e.g. fever and pain) and where successful treatment of the bladder with antibiotics will be followed by the disappearance of associated symptoms of incontinence and urgency. On the other hand, the urinary infection may indicate a *chronic bacteriuria*, which itself may be secondary to underlying disease within the bladder or of the neurological control of the bladder. These may be associated with a degree of residual urine. In such a case the symptoms of incontinence are those of the underlying cause of bladder dysfunction, and the infection is secondary. Elimination of the infection will not then affect the symptoms. In this case there is almost certain to be recurrence of the infection, either with the same or with a different organism, within a matter of weeks or months.

It is not always easy to distinguish between these two types of infection and if there is any doubt then a course of the appropriate antibiotic should be given as a therapeutic trial.

In summary, a urinary infection is occasionally the cause of incontinence. More often the infection is a chronic bacteriuria and both it, and the incontinence, are evidence of another underlying pathology.

*Impairment of the neurological control of micturition*

This is the most important cause of incontinence in old people. Its full understanding requires an appreciation of how the young baby acquires control of micturition. A simplified account of this is as follows.

In the young child the bladder fills from the kidneys and as it becomes distended its stretch-receptors are activated. These discharge impulses through the afferent autonomic nerves to the second, third and fourth sacral segments of the spinal cord. In this area, through the various interneurones, the physiological mechanisms of recruitment and after-discharge lead to the activation of efferent impulses. These pass, from time to time, through the parasympathetic nerves causing small intrinsic contractions of the bladder wall. As the bladder becomes more distended these contractions become more frequent until a very large one occurs which causes the bladder to empty. This emptying is reflex and the baby is therefore incontinent (see Fig. 8.3).

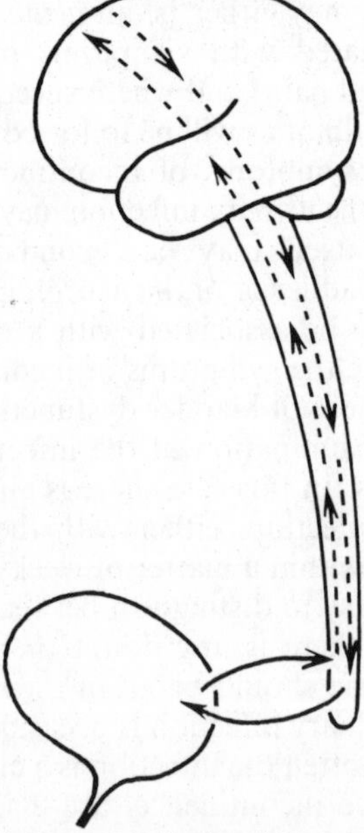

Fig. 8.3 The neurological control of micturition.

As time goes by the young child learns first of all to appreciate in consciousness the sensation of bladder distension by developing pathways through the posterior columns of the spinal cord to an area of the frontal cortex lying within the cingulate gyrus. At the same time the child becomes aware of the social desirability of acquiring continence (that, for instance, its mother is pleased when it empties its bladder in the appropriate receptacle, and is likely to be displeased when it allows its bladder to empty inappropriately). The young child, therefore, sends down through the developing, long tracts in the lateral parts of the spinal cord impulses which block the reflex arc at the 'sacral bladder centre'. These are *inhibitory* impulses since they effectively inhibit the genesis of intrinsic bladder contractions. Once the child has learnt to inhibit these its bladder will fill up without emptying itself reflexly. When time and place are appropriate for micturition he can stop inhibiting and indeed can facilitate bladder contractions, at the same time relaxing the striated muscles of the pelvic diaphragm, and also deliberately increasing the intra-abdominal pressure. He will then micturate consciously. Once this neurological process has been acquired it normally stays with the individual throughout life. The bladder of the normal adult shows no intrinsic contractions until voluntary emptying begins.

This is a complex process which may be interrupted at a number of different levels within the central nervous system. The different lesions which cause such disruptions cause the various types of the *neurogenic* (or neuropathic) *bladder*.

The simplest *classification of the neurogenic bladder* is into four groups: the autonomous, the atonic, the reflex and the uninhibited (Fig. 8.4).

*The autonomous neurogenic bladder*

The autonomous neurogenic bladder occurs when the bladder centre in the sacral cord is destroyed and the bladder is completely decentralized. This happens in spina bifida and very occasionally in people who have tumours of the cauda equina, or who have vascular damage to the lower end of the spinal cord. In this case the bladder will be quite devoid of conscious sensation. It will fill and empty inefficiently and

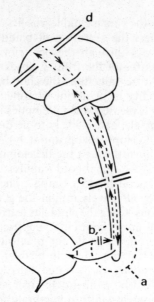

Fig. 8.4 Classification of the neurogenic bladder. *Key:* a, autonomous; b, atonic; c, reflex; d, uninhibited.

automatically as a result of single axonal reflexes and other reflex activity through the peripheral nerves. The patient will therefore be incontinent.

*The atonic neurogenic bladder*

Here, there is disease affecting the posterior nerve roots or the posterior horn cells. The sensation of bladder distension is lost although cortical voluntary inhibition is retained. This is the typical bladder of tabes dorsalis and of diabetic autonomic neuropathy. Because the person is unaware of bladder distension, the bladder becomes over distended from time to time, and gradually becomes chronically atonic. This leads to *chronic retention with overflow incontinence.*

*The reflex neurogenic bladder*

This is the bladder which results from a lesion above the sacral bladder centre affecting both afferent and efferent fibres. This occurs most commonly with transection of the spinal

cord commonly due to motorcycle, motor car or riding accidents or in some patients with multiple sclerosis, in whom the
demyelinating plaques affect both these tracts. It is, therefore,
the bladder of the paraplegic and it is identical with the
bladder of the baby. There is neither sensation of bladder
distension nor the ability to inhibit intrinsic bladder contractions, and so bladder emptying is reflex and the patient is
incontinent. Occasionally paraplegics learn to fire off intrinsic
bladder contractions at a time which is suitable to them by
stimulating the skin within the second, third and fourth sacral
dermatomes.

*The uninhibited neurogenic bladder*

Here the sensation of bladder distension is retained but the
power to inhibit is lost and this is typically due to a lesion in
the cerebral cortex. It most commonly occurs in patients with
cerebrovascular disease, including some with stroke and
occasionally with cerebral tumour. Some impairment of the
cortical bladder centre results from aging within the neurones
of the cerebral cortex. Just as memory impairment, an increase
in sway, some impairment of the control of the vasomotor
function and thermoregulation may be accompaniments of
aging of the brain, so some degree of the uninhibited neurogenic bladder may be present also for this reason.

The uninhibited neurogenic bladder may be present without
causing incontinence, but with the symptoms of nocturnal
frequency and urgency. Since sensation is retained the feeling
of desire to void often occurs when intravesical pressure rises
in association with an uninhibited contraction: since this contraction may quickly lead to bladder emptying the patient
suffers from urgency. This type of incontinence is sometimes
therefore described as *'urge incontinence'*.

In old people the uninhibited neurogenic bladder is often a
predisposing cause or *predisposing factor* causing impairment
of bladder control which can be compensated for by adjusting
the environment to suit the badly-functioning bladder. Thus a
bedside commode or nearby lavatory allow the person with
nocturnal frequency and urgency to empty the bladder
safely. Such a patient may also curtail journeys out during the
day to those which her badly-functioning bladder can cope

with. She may not, therefore, become incontinent unless some additional *precipitating factor* comes along. Usually this is something which robs her of her independence, and so makes her dependent on other people: they in their turn may not realize how her bladder works and how she needs to empty it quickly once the sensation of bladder distension arises. Common precipitating factors are: becoming bedfast due to an acute infection (e.g. chest infection) or due to trauma (e.g. fracture of the femur); occasionally a change of environment so that the old person wakes up bewildered in the night, not knowing where the toilet is, and occasionally it is the effect of factors which produce an acute confusional disorder (e.g. drugs or toxic or anoxic factors) which further impair the cortical bladder centre.

Probably the commonest situation is when an old woman is admitted to hospital and the night nurse does not realize that normally she gets up two or three times during the night at home to empty her bladder. Unless the night nurse will help her to do this quickly in hospital then her bladder will inevitably empty itself and she will be incontinent. It is therefore important that all hospital beds should be adjustable in their height to allow elderly patients to have the bed low at night with a bedside commode, and to get out to the commode with the minimum of help whenever necessary. All nurses looking after geriatric patients should realize the implications of the uninhibited neurogenic bladder in the elderly.

*Diagnosis.* The uninhibited neurogenic bladder can often be diagnosed from the history: evidence of cerebrovascular disease will support such a diagnosis. However, the diagnosis can only be made confidently by carrying out a *cystometrogram* and this simple investigation should be undertaken whenever there is any doubt.

A *cystometrogram* is simply a method of observing (and recording) the reaction of the bladder to increasing distension. The bladder is filled from a reservoir through a two-way catheter, the other tube of the two-way catheter being connected to a manometer and usually through that to a recording device. Often the manometer is omitted and a transducer used to convert changes in fluid pressure to a recording on paper. In carrying out a cystometrogram the bladder may either be filled in increments of 50 ml at a time from the reservoir, or it may be filled gradually and continuously in drops. The most physiological method is to allow the bladder to fill of its own accord from the secretion of urine, but this is much too time-consuming to be practical. The method of incremental filling, while it is unphysiological, has the advantage of allowing a standardized technique in which the bladder's reaction to distension at a constant rate may be noted.

The cystometrogram allows the following measurements to be recorded:

1. Residual urine
2. Resting intravesical pressure
3. Bladder capacity
4. Intravesical pressure throughout filling and at the point of emptying
5. The point at which desire to void is first felt
6. The presence and timing of any uninhibited contractions and whether or not they lead to bladder emptying.

Additional information may be obtained by getting the patient to attempt to micturate or by noting the effect of certain provocative stimuli such as movement, coughing etc.. All types of the uninhibited neurogenic bladder may be diagnosed by cystometrogram, as shown in Figure 8.5.

*Management.* Treatment of the uninhibited neurogenic bladder is by the use of drugs which substitute a pharmacological blockade in the reflex arc of micturition for the neurogenic inhibition which has been lost. Such drugs are usually the antimuscarine type of anticholinergics and they include *atropine* and the solanaceous alkaloids (belladonna), *propantheline, emepronium bromide, flavoxate* and indeed drugs with any anticholinergic effect which are used for other purposes such as the antiparkinsonian drugs (e.g. orphenadrine and the tricyclic antidepressants (imipramine). All these block neurotransmission, either in the peripheral autonomic ganglia or at the motor end plate in the bladder muscle; thus they diminish the genesis of uninhibited contractions, allowing bladder capacity to be increased. One problem with these drugs is that they can also increase residual urine, by promoting a tendency to chronic retention (and, of course, retention of urine is an

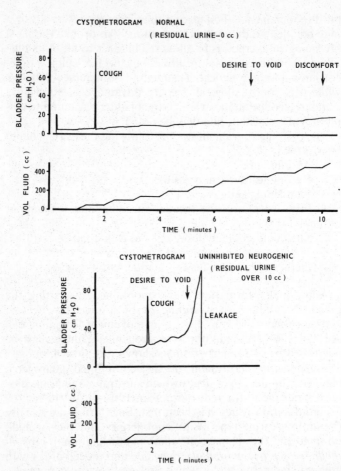

Fig. 8.5 Cystometrogram patterns (upper figure=normal; lower=uninhibited neurogenic).

occasional unwanted side effect when the drugs are being used for other purposes).

The *time of administration* of these drugs: if the patient is incontinent only at night (as is often the case) then the medication should be given before she retires to bed (e.g. at 10 p.m.) and again when she wakens up during the night to empty her bladder (e.g. at 2 a.m.) and need not be given at any other time. If the patient is living alone then it may be necessary for her to set an alarm clock to waken herself during the night. On the other hand, if the incontinence is present throughout the day then the drug should be given six hourly. In short they should be given at a time to anticipate the episode of wetting.

The anticholinergics most widely used at the present time are emepronium bromide (Cetiprin) 200 mg at a time, and flavoxate (Urispas) 200 mg. Combinations (e.g. propantheline and orphenadrine) have also been used with success. Drugs of this type will in many cases make all the difference between continence and incontinence, but they are obviously no substitute for the ready and regular access of the patient to a lavatory. They should be given a trial of about four weeks and if not successful they should not be persisted with.

Recently another group of drugs the beta-adrenergic stimulating drugs have been introduced into the management of the uninhibited neurogenic bladder. *Orciprenaline* has been suggested for use in combination with emepronium bromide or flavoxate.

*The unstable bladder*

This is impairment of bladder control without any obvious lesion within the central nervous system. The presenting features are also different. Bladder emptying is triggered off by a physical stimulus, such as the patient coughing or getting up from bed or chair. The condition is distinguished from stress incontinence because in the latter the rise in intravesical pressure on coughing or moving, overcomes a weak bladder outlet and squeezes out a small amount of urine. In the unstable bladder the stimulus leads to an immediate uninhibited bladder contraction with emptying of most or all of the bladder contents.

The unstable bladder can also be distinguished on the cystometrogram because no contractions arise during normal filling, but a provocative stimulus (cough, movement, running in cold water) causes an uninhibited contraction which can be seen.

Management is by anticholinergic drugs. Flavoxate is often used in this condition.

## The practical management of incontinence

Once a diagnosis has been made and specific treatment applied the majority of cases of urinary incontinence will be controlled. Occasionally, however, patients with intractable incontinence present in whom no treatment is successful. This is particularly the case in patients with arterio-sclerotic dementia. In these cases consideration must then be given to the use of pads, appliances and catheters.

*Incontinence pads*

Many large incontinence pads are on the market for use on beds or chairs. These contain material which absorbs liquid and they have a waterproof backing. Unfortunately they remain wet as the patient lies or sits on them and may thus lead to the formation of urine rashes on the skin. Also with any quantity of urine they tend to form a lake and the urine may run off the edge of the pad, wetting the bed. However, as a method of protection of bedding against occasional wetting they have a place.

There are two incontinence pads designed to be worn on the person which are effective in certain situations: the Gelling pad and the Marsupial pad.

*Gelling pad.* This is a sanitary pad which contains in the centre a powdered methyl cellulose together with a deodorant.

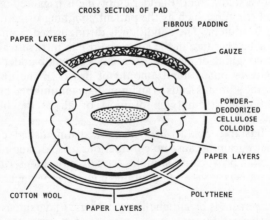

Fig. 8.6 The Gelling Pad.

It is covered on its upper surface by a non-wettable polyurethane net and on the lower surface by a waterproof backing (see Fig. 8.6). It is worn as a sanitary pad and when urine is passed it forms a jelly with the powdered cellulose. Thus the skin is kept dry and because of the deodorant there is no smell. This pad is particularly useful in patients with stress incontinence or occasional incontinence who may pass up to 50 or 100 ml of urine at a time. It can absorb about 250 ml of urine altogether but will not do this if it is all passed at once, and therefore it is not necessarily successful in patients with uninhibited neurogenic incontinence.

*Marsupial pad.* The Marsupial pad is worn in a special pair of close-fitting pants ('Kanga Pants') containing a pouch so that the pad can be inserted into this pouch from the front (Fig. 8.7). It is separated from the skin by a layer of non-

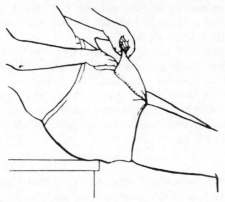

Fig. 8.7 The Marsupial Pad.

wettable polyurethane mesh. If these pants are properly fitted they also provide useful protection against occasional wetting.

*Appliances*

Various appliances have been produced to be worn in the management of incontinence and these must be considered separately for each sex.

*Males.* Different types of penile clamps are available but their use is extremely limited and in particular they are contra-indicated for patients with uninhibited neurogenic bladders, since anything which obstructs the outflow of urine during the uninhibited contractions will raise still further the intravesical pressure encouraging the formation of bladder diverticula and of ureteral reflux. Many appliances to be worn over the penis have been produced. The simplest of these is a length of *Paul's tubing* which is particularly useful with men who are bedfast because of paralysis or coma and who are incontinent. A number of *sheath urinals* have been produced which act in a similar fashion.

Of all the other more elaborate urinals probably the only one which is reasonably successful is the pubic pressure urinal. Here a ring is worn encircling the base of the penis and strapped firmly against the pubis. Onto this ring is fixed a beak-shaped device which encloses the penis and which leads into a bag worn on the leg. The *pubic pressure urinal* is useful for men who are mobile and incontinent. Care must be taken to see that it fits accurately and that it does not become either kinked or the bag over-filled.

Unfortunately, most aged men with intractable incontinence are also quite intolerant of such appliances and will interfere with them or indeed pull them off. However in younger patients, particularly paraplegics, they are often more useful.

*Females.* Although a variety of portable urinals has been marketed for use with females there is none which is successful at the present time.

### Catheters

If all other methods of treatment of urinary incontinence fail then the use of an indwelling catheter to be worn permanently is the final method of control. For this purpose, Foley catheters (retained in the bladder by an inflatable balloon) are used and they are worn attached to a collecting bag which is worn on the leg. On no account should an indwelling catheter be worn with a bag which either lies on the floor or is attached to the furniture, since not only is this degrading for the patient but it serves also as an anchor to immobilize him. Leg bags should have a flutter valve incorporated into them so that they may be worn also when the patient is lying in bed (Fig. 8.8). Patients can usually be taught to empty the bag themselves every four or six hours. In addition to the standard Foley

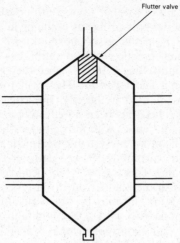

Fig. 8.8 A leg bag.

catheter there is now produced the Silastic catheter. This has a special coating which prevents adherence of salts and debris, It is claimed that the Silastic catheter can be worn for a period of three to six months without changing. The regular Foley catheter will need changing usually every fortnight.

One drawback about indwelling catheterization is that it is inevitably accompanied by infection of the urine. Bacteria will ascend not only within the catheter but also in the film between the catheter and the urethra. While it is possible to maintain a sterile closed system of catheter drainage for a few days it is not practicable to do this for longer periods, particularly in patients who are mobile. Therefore, infection of the urine has to be accepted as an inevitable feature of indwelling catheterization.

Fortunately, such infection appears to be benign in as much as it does not produce systemic effects. In the short term (i.e. a period of two to five years) it seems to produce no serious effects on the kidney. Since the life expectancy of most patients with intractable incontinence who may require indwelling catheterization is likely to be in the region of two years the risks of infection can be quite reasonably accepted, particularly if by the use of an indwelling catheter it is possible for the old person to remain dry rather than continuously wet for these last years, and possibly to live at home or in an old persons' home rather than in a long-stay hospital ward.

It is not usual practice to give antibiotics systemically in patients with indwelling catheters since they will sterilize the urine only for a short period. They will produce resistent organisms and, if used frequently, side-effects become very real problems. There has been no effective assessment of the use of urinary antiseptics with indwelling catheters and at the present time, therefore, no systemic treatment is normally used unless an acute infection occurs (a catheter fever producing pyrexia and pain). This is a very rare occurrence. It is usual, however, to wash the bladder out from time to time with an antiseptic solution. This may best be done after changing the catheter (i.e. every two weeks). Sixty millilitres of a solution such as 2 per cent neomycin or one in 5000 cetrimide is instilled into the bladder through the new catheter: this is clamped for half an hour, then it is drained and the whole thing washed out with 2 litres of normal saline.

FURTHER READING

Caldwell, K.P.S. (Ed.) (1975) *Urinary Incontinence*. London: Sector Publishing Limited.

# 9. Faecal Incontinence

Faecal incontinence is often thought of as an unhappy but inevitable association with old age. However, as with pressure sores, it might more appropriately be regarded as a failure of medical and nursing management for with proper diagnosis and treatment, faecal incontinence in old people is almost entirely preventable. Its importance lies not only in the unpleasant and degrading situation in which the patient finds himself, but also in the fact that it may be a symptom of serious and possibly treatable disease of the lower bowel. Clinically faecal incontinence may present in two ways: in the first place as frequent and, indeed, almost constant soiling with semi-formed faeces, and in the second place as the passage of a formed stool once or twice a day into the bed or into the clothing. These different methods of presentation have different causes and are clues as to the diagnosis. Causes of faecal incontinence may be divided into three groups (see Table 9.1):

Table 9.1 Causes of faecal incontinence

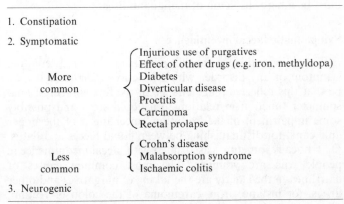

1. Constipation

2. Symptomatic

More common
- Injurious use of purgatives
- Effect of other drugs (e.g. iron, methyldopa)
- Diabetes
- Diverticular disease
- Proctitis
- Carcinoma
- Rectal prolapse

Less common
- Crohn's disease
- Malabsorption syndrome
- Ischaemic colitis

3. Neurogenic

1. That due to constipation
2. That which is symptomatic of underlying disease affecting the large bowel
3. That which is due to the impairment of the neurological control of defaecation.

## Faecal incontinence due to constipation

This is almost certainly the commonest cause of faecal incontinence in the elderly and is particularly common in long-stay geriatric hospitals because of its association with physical disability and immobility. The diagnosis is made both on the history and also on rectal examination. The characteristic clinical pattern is of unformed or semi-formed stools being found many times a day: the patient is almost constantly soiled. Faecal impaction by hard masses is a common cause, but constipation with a rectum filled with firm but not hard faeces may also be associated with faecal incontinence. Once the diagnosis has been made treatment should be instituted as described on p. 153 and then steps taken to ensure that the condition, once cured, does not return. If incontinence remains after constipation has been successfully treated, then a full investigation must be carried out to discover a cause for it within the lower alimentary tract and in this situation there must be a high suspicion of malignant disease.

## Symptomatic faecal incontinence

Faecal incontinence in old people may be a presenting symptom of any disorder which produces *diarrhoea*. It may be that this reflects an age change in the fine control of anal sphincter function in relation to a liquid stool and possibly some impairment of the 'sampling' mechanism of the upper anal canal for distinguishing between liquid faeces and flatus. Diarrhoea is sometimes associated with faecal incontinence in people who are younger. The most common causes of diarrhoea in the elderly are the taking of purgatives and other drugs, for instance iron, carcinoma of the colon or rectum, diverticular disease, simple granular proctitis, ulcerative colitis, ischaemic colitis or gastroenteritis. All of these indicate the need for proper investigation, including sigmoidoscopy and barium enema.

Other occasional causes of symptomatic faecal incontinence are diabetes, thyrotoxicosis, prolapse of the rectum and disruption of the anal sphincter (e.g. in an incompetent operation for haemorrhoids). The treatment is that of the underlying disorder and if this is untreatable then symptomatic treatment of faecal incontinence is as that described below for neurogenic incontinence.

## Neurogenic faecal incontinence

The normal process of defaecation follows a gastrocolic reflex. This causes movement of a faecal mass from the descending colon into the rectum. This rectal distension is followed by relaxation of the internal sphincter and by intrinsic contractions of the rectum itself. In the normal person, if defaecation is not possible, then the act is postponed by the voluntary inhibition of the rectal contractions and a rapid return of the contracting tone to the internal sphincter. In the elderly, however, and particularly in patients suffering from cerebrovascular disease, the ability to postpone the act of defaecation may be impaired or lost. This may be demonstrated by distending a balloon in the rectum and noting whether this leads to a series of intrinsic contractions followed by the involuntary passage of the balloon (Fig. 9.1) or whether the

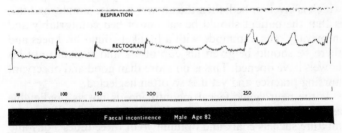

Fig. 9.1 Rectogram.

rectum accepts the distending mass without showing any intrinsic contractions (Fig. 9.2). In the latter case, the reflex arc arising from stretch receptors in the rectum is inhibited by a voluntary (although eventually subconscious) process. In the

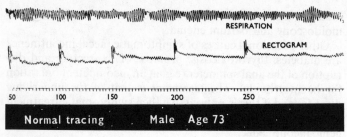

RESPIRATION

RECTOGRAM

50    100    150    200    250

**Normal tracing    Male    Age 73**

Fig. 9.2 Rectogram.

former case, the contractions are uninhibited and lead to incontinent passage of formed or semi-formed stools.

This type of incontinence is seen most characteristically in patients who have multiple cerebral infarcts or who suffer from arteriosclerotic dementia. Whether or not it also occurs as a result of age change within the central and peripheral nervous systems themselves is still a matter of debate.

The clinical picture therefore is of one or two formed stools found in the bed or clothing each day and these usually follow meals or hot beverages.

*Management* (see Fig. 9.3)

The management of this condition is to try and prevent the reflex emptying of the colon following rectal distension and to secure bowel motions under controlled conditions. If the incontinent stool is passed following an early morning cup of tea which is given in bed, then the answer is quite simple, and this is that the patient should be sat out of bed comfortably and in privacy on a commode with a blanket round his knees and there he should be given his cup of tea and remain until his bowels have opened. This is no more than good and observant nursing practice and yet it is so often neglected.

If the neurogenic faecal incontinence is not as predictable as this, then it may be controlled by giving a constipating mixture such as chalk and opium two or three times a day and securing bowel evacuation under controlled conditions by giving an enema or suppositories once or twice a week. This régime needs careful individual adjustment.

In conclusion, it cannot be overemphasized that persistent faecal incontinence in old people is a failure of medical and

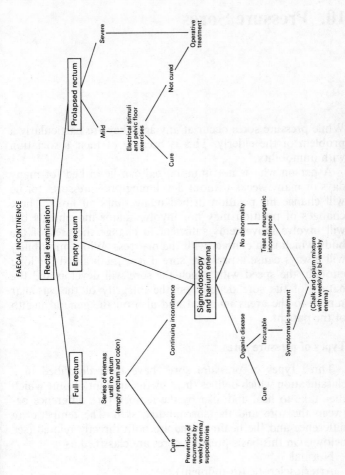

Fig. 9.3 Flow diagram of the diagnosis of faecal incontinence.

nursing practice. It is a matter which must be taken seriously by both doctors and nurses. It is not a normal accompaniment of old age and it may be the first evidence of serious and treatable disease within the bowel.

# 10. Pressure Sores

While pressure sores occur at any age, they are particularly a problem of the elderly. This is because of their association with immobility.

A person who is not immobilized can lie in bed for many days or many weeks without developing pressure sores for he will change his position in bed many times an hour. These changes of position may not involve major movements but will involve movements sufficient to change the area of the body which is in contact with the mattress. While immobility will always cause a pressure sore if it is maintained for long enough, the speed with which the sore will develop and the nature of the sore depend on the integrity of the vascular supply to the areas involved and also on the general health of the patient.

**Types of pressure sores**

Three types of pressure sores have been described in a classification which defines them by the amount of time which they take to heal and also by the temperature difference between the sore and the surrounding skin. The temperature difference and the healing time are both directly related (see below). On this basis pressure sores are classified as:

Normal

Arteriosclerotic (or indolent)

Terminal

*Normal* pressure sores will heal within about six weeks and there is a temperature difference of less than $2.5°C$ between the area of the sore and the area of the surrounding skin. In other words, the blood supply is intact and the sore has been produced entirely by ischaemia due to pressure.

*Arteriosclerotic* ulcers take about 16 weeks to heal*: there is a temperature difference of at least 1°C between the area of the ulcer and surrounding skin. This indicates that impairment of blood supply due to vascular disease has contributed to the development of the sore, as well as pressure.

*Terminal* ulcers occur in people who are dying and do not heal.

## Types of pressure

Two types of pressure contribute to the development of pressure sores—compression and shearing forces. A third element, not a form of pressure but rather distortion of the skin, is skin folding.

### Compression

On the well-known law that a force which is applied to a solid object will produce an equal and opposite force, we may examine what happens to the human body as it lies flat on a variety of different surfaces. This is illustrated in Fig. 10.1 which indicates that the area of the body coming into contact with the surface depends on the malleability of the surface lain on. A body lying on a wooden or concrete floor will be in contact with that surface in only certain areas and the whole force from the mass of the body will be distributed to the floor through those few areas. Thus the pressure in these areas will be large. The opposite force will be equally large and the resulting compression of the soft tissues lying between the bony skeleton and the hard surface will be considerable. At the other extreme we may consider a body lying on a water-containing mattress where the whole area of the under-surface of the body is in contact with the surface of the mattress. In this case the weight of the body is distributed over a much larger area, so the force at any particular part of the body surface is a great deal less and the compression of the soft tissues is correspondingly less (Fig. 10.1). What is critical to the development of pressure sores is whether the compressing force is greater than the pressure of blood within the arterioles

---

*The economics of pressure sores: unnecessary hospitalisation for 16 weeks at £60 per week = £1000.

AREA OF SUPPORT VARIES WITH NATURE OF SUPPORTING SURFACE

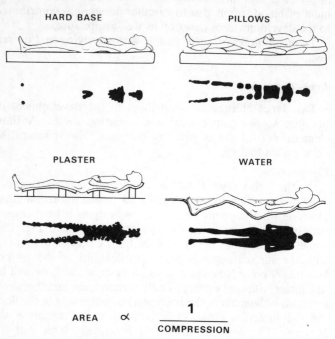

Fig. 10.1 Area of the body in contact with various surfaces. (After Lowthian.)

and capillaries. The capillary blood pressure is 33 mm Hg at the arteriolar end and 16 mm Hg at the venous end. If the compressing force is less than this, the skin will remain intact even if the person lies immobile for long periods of time. This is the case with the complete water-bed or for someone lying on a perfectly moulded hard surface such as a plaster cast. An ingenious experiment carried out to assess the compressive force of the body, used a bed of nails (heads up) each attached to a spring and to a measuring device. Pressure in the sacral area was 60 to 70 mm Hg and over the heels 30 to 45 mm Hg.

*Shearing forces*

Many bedfast patients do not lie flat but are supported in

## SHEARING FORCE

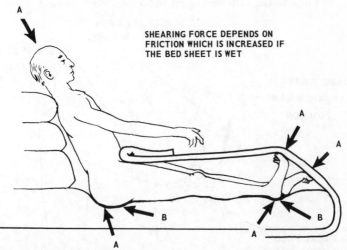

SHEARING FORCE DEPENDS ON
FRICTION WHICH IS INCREASED IF
THE BED SHEET IS WET

Fig. 10.2 Shearing forces. A=compressing force; B=shearing force. (After Lowthian.)

various semi-recumbent positions as shown in Figure 10.2. There is then a tendency of the body to slide forward until it would come to lie flat. This tendency can only be counteracted by either some obstruction to the forward movement of the body (such as the feet coming to the end of the bed) or a high coefficient of friction between the body and the surface on which it lies (tending to make the body adhere to this surface). In this case it is the skin which will adhere, while the bony skeleton will tend to continue moving forward and produce lines of stress in subcutaneous tissues. These are called shearing forces and they may do two things: they may obstruct the small arteries and arterioles by distorting them or they may even rupture them.

### Folding

In addition to the shearing forces, movement of the body on the surface on which it is lying with adherence of the skin to the surface may produce actual folds in the skin itself. This is more likely to happen in emaciated individuals in whom the skin is lax and will only occur in those areas where the skin is not closely adherent to the bony skeleton (see Fig. 10.3). Folding of the skin will again obliterate blood vessels.

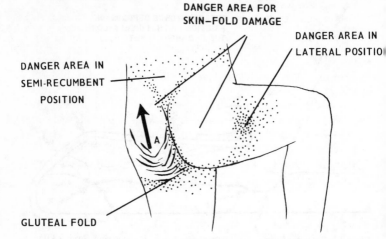

Fig. 10.3 Areas where skin folding may occur. (After Lowthian.)

These then are the causes of ischaemia. The next important factor is to discover how long ischaemia may be continued before it leads to necrosis. Animal experiments, for instance, occluding the circulation in rabbit's ears (at 100 mm Hg), have shown that: 2 hours compression → no significant lesion seen 2 days later; 7 hours compression → tissue oedema and blood extravasation for the next 18 hours, endothelial damage still apparent 12 days later.

In addition to the direct ischaemic effects of compression and folding there must be added the results of endothelial cell damage, platelet clumping and oedema. All tend to produce tissue necrosis.

*Summary*

Compression causes ischaemia and this will be most apparent when the body is lying on a surface which does not fit its contours.

Shearing forces cause ischaemia which will be most in evidence where there is a high degree of friction between the body and the surface lain on (especially if there is wetting between these two surfaces).

Folding causes ischaemia, and this will be most severe in emaciated individuals.

Immobility is the basic underlying factor.

The surface on which the body lies, by greater or lesser distribution of compressing force, will increase or diminish it at any one place.

The semirecumbent position together with the coefficient of friction of the material on which the body lies (which will be increased by incontinence) contributes to the shearing force.

Emaciation contributes to the degree of skin folding.

General health and adequacy of vascular sufficiency are also contributory.

Treatment and prevention of pressure sores must depend on measures designed to affect these various phenomena.

## Prevention

In theory the prevention of pressure sores is quite simple. Patients who are at risk should be identified and compression, shearing and folding effects prevented. Those at risk are the immobile, particularly those:

in coma
in pain (post operative or in hip or knee joint)
with heavy plasters
paralysed
with Parkinsonism.

Secondary factors include:
emaciation
incontinence
poor general state.

One satisfactory system of identifying patients at risk is to use a scoring system such as that shown in Figure 10.4. This chart should be completed by the doctor as he admits the patient. A score below 12 indicates a patient at risk. He should

COLOUR CARD ASSESSMENT

| Name of Patient: | | | | |
|---|---|---|---|---|
| Unit No. | | | | |
| | | | Date | |
| | marks | | | |
| **GENERAL PYHSICAL CONDITION:** | | | | |
| Good | 4 | | | |
| Fair | 3 | | | |
| Poor | 2 | | | |
| Very bad | 1 | | | |
| **MENTAL STATE:** | | | | |
| Alert | 4 | | | |
| Apathetic | 3 | | | |
| Confused | 2 | | | |
| Stuporose | 1 | | | |
| **ACTIVITY:** | | | | |
| Ambulant | 4 | | | |
| Ambulant with help | 3 | | | |
| Chairbound | 2 | | | |
| Confined to bed | 1 | | | |
| **MOBILITY:** | | | | |
| Full | 4 | | | |
| Slightly limited | 3 | | | |
| Very limited | 2 | | | |
| Immobile | 1 | | | |
| **INCONTINENCE:** | | | | |
| Not incontinent | 4 | | | |
| Occasionally incontinent | 3 | | | |
| Usually incontinent of urine | 2 | | | |
| Doubly incontinent | 1 | | | |
| | Total | | | |

Fig. 10.4 At risk chart.

immediately receive special attention from nurses including:
    Alternating pressure mattress
    Some additional protection for the heels (see below—Tubeypads, sheepskin pads)
    A bed cradle.

*Overcoming immobility*

Immobility can be prevented by changing the position of the patient on the surface on which he is lying from time to time by some external agency. The frequency with which this ought to be done will depend on the nature of the surface on which he lies. The custom was for the nursing staff to lift him into a new position every hour or two. This is the traditional way of preventing pressure sores but it has its limitations. These are:

1. It is expensive in nursing time
2. It is disturbing to the patient, particularly if movements are painful.

Various methods of moving the surface rather than the patient have been introduced, for instance, a bed which tilts itself from side to side mechanically, but the only really effective method is the alternating pressure mattress. The mattress

## RIPPLE MATTRESS

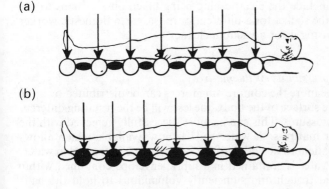

**INFLATE BEFORE PATIENT GOES ON IT**

**WATCH FOR FAILURE**

**AS RECUMBENT AS POSSIBLE**

Fig. 10.5 Alternating pressure mattress.

(sometimes known as the 'ripple bed') is arranged so that each alternate tube is inflated simultaneously. Thus when all the tubes arrowed in Figure 10.5 (a) are inflated, the compressing forces are shown and when, a few minutes later these are deflated and the tubes arrowed in Fig. 10.5 (b) are inflated, the area of compression moves to a different part. Thus no area of skin is subject to continuous compression for more than whatever time is decided by the cycle of the pump. In the 'Frustro-Conical Alternating Pressure Mattress' the tubes have a diameter of 11·5 centimetres and the pump cycle is 7 minutes. The alternating pressure mattress marks a great advance in the prevention of pressure sores; however, it has some limitations of its own, such as:

1. It is a machine, and subject both to mechanical failure and to human error in its use. The former is signalled by a warning light but this must be seen and acted upon by the nursing staff.

2. The pump may fail for various reasons which may include the electric plug being taken out, perhaps to use the socket for a different purpose, e.g. a domestic worker using it for a vacuum cleaner.

*Compressibility of the mattress*

The more the compressing forces can be distributed over the whole surface of the body, the less will be the resulting differential pressures. This can be most successfully achieved with the water mattress. A water-bed* is now available which allows the patient to lie with half the body surface immersed in water. The water is contained in a fabric envelope contained within a rigid trough and sufficiently voluminous to hold the half-submerged body. There is a heating element to maintain the temperature of the water.

The main difficulty with the water-bed is the nursing of the patient and it is not suitable for patients who are incontinent. It is also difficult for patients to get in and out of and may, therefore, tend to increase the period of bedfastness. If this is

*The Beaufort-Winchester Flotation Bed.

avoided by getting the patient out on to his feet each day, the water-bed can be very successful in both preventing and healing pressure sores.

*Preventing shearing forces*

Shearing forces can be prevented either by sitting patients out of bed or lying them flat in bed. The risk is also increased when patients lie in wet beds, thereby increasing the coefficient of friction. If the patients have to be nursed in the erect sitting position, then it may be helpful to arrange the bed with a board at the foot to prevent shearing. A cradle should always be used to protect the feet of elderly patients from the pressure of the bedclothing. Sheepskins and artificial sheepskins will help to prevent shearing without causing a high degree of friction, they will slightly disseminate compressing forces but they will not eliminate them. Sheepskins, however, are very comfortable for thin and emaciated patients to lie on and may quite properly be used on top of the ripple mattress.

*Special equipment for the prevention of sores on the heels*

This includes Tubey-gauze (a form of stretch gauze with a foam rubber inset which can be fitted over the foot and prevent direct contact between the bed and the heel) and also sheepskin heel pads. Both of these will eliminate friction and shearing forces but neither will prevent compressing forces. They are useful aids, but will not in themselves prevent the development of pressure sores on the heels.

Another method of keeping pressure off the heels is to put a Lennard pad (a wedge-shaped foam pad, contoured to the shape of the calf) under the leg, so that the heel itself is kept free of the bed. This pad may also be wrapped around the leg. A similar effect is produced by using pillows under the legs. This may be more satisfactory since the pillows can be extended right up to the buttocks. Any form of compression of the calves may cause venous thrombosis but if the support is spread under the whole of the leg (as with pillows properly placed) then this liability will be minimized.

## The treatment of established pressure sores

The methods discussed above for the prevention of pressure sores should, of course, be instigated at once if a pressure sore is present and, if it is severe, the use of a water-bed should be considered.

The next matter is to get rid of infection which can usually be done by local dressings of eusol, cetrimide or other antiseptic. Systemic antibiotics need only be used if there is an area of surrounding cellulitis.

Then there may remain a black eschar of necrotic tissue and healing will not proceed until this has been removed. Very often it takes a long time before this eschar separates if left to itself; the process may be hastened by surgical removal or by the application of various substances of which perhaps the most useful is 'Trypure'. This is a trypsin preparation which can be either sprinkled on as a powder and covered with a saline dressing, or more satisfactorily may be injected through a small hypodermic needle a few drops at a time around the edge of the eschar, beneath the dead tissue.

Once the sore is sterile and free of eschar, healing will proceed naturally at a rate dependent on whether it is a 'normal' ulcer or an arteriosclerotic ('indolent') ulcer (see above). Very often the period of healing can be accelerated by the use of plastic surgery. The plastic surgeon should be called in consultation as soon as the eschar has separated and infection cleared.

Many other methods have been suggested as accelerating the healing of pressure sores and these divide themselves into:

Substances taken systemically
Those applied locally.

General measures include the correction of anaemia. In moderately severe anaemia a blood transfusion may accelerate healing. There is very good evidence that administration of ascorbic acid by mouth accelerates wound healing in the pressure sore. There is less convincing evidence that the taking of zinc sulphate (120 mg in a capsule) also accelerates the healing of pressure sores. It does appear that many patients with pressure sores have low plasma zinc levels. Anabolic steroids have also been suggested in the past but there is no evidence that they accelerate healing.

As far as local therapy is concerned, a vast range of substances has been tried empirically at one time or another—

from marmalade to chlorophyll and from oxygen to insulin.
One of these is the application of ultraviolet light and there is
some evidence that this may have an effect. There is no good
evidence for any of the other substances that have been used.

In the case of deep and especially undermined pressure sores,
it has been the custom to pack them with ribbon gauze, soaked
in Eusol. An alternative method of treatment is to pack them
with honey which has the advantage of being an osmotic
antiseptic and at the same time non-abrasive and having the
effect of a fluid cushion.

# 11. Bone Disease and Fractures

Three kinds of bone disease are common in old people: osteoporosis, osteomalacia and Paget's disease ('osteitis deformans'). All three give rise to bone pains and predispose to fracture, but they are different in their basic nature. The first two are disorders of bone metabolism, and therefore generalized, though with local variations in intensity. Osteitis deformans is a localized or diffuse but never generalized disease of unknown origin.

## Osteoporosis

Osteoporosis remains an enigma in spite of much probing of its cause. A few solid facts about it have, however, been established.

> 1. *The fundamental change is reduction of the total amount of bone in the skeleton*
> 2. The histology of affected bone is normal. So is analysis of the chemical content after ashing, though this is a comparatively crude method which would not reveal possibly important nuances of molecular structure
> 3. The serum calcium and phosphorous concentrations and the serum alkaline phosphatase level of activity are normal.

Measurements of the total amount of bone at various ages in a large cross-section of the population have shewn an increase up to the age of 30; the total bone content then remains constant till about age 45, after which it falls progressively in both sexes, but more precipitately after the menopause in women.

Osteoporosis is then a 'physiological' effect of advancing age, and 'clinical' osteoporosis only emerges when total bone is reduced below some critical level at which fractures are more likely to occur and the bones become painful when stressed. There is suggestive evidence that those who have an above average amount of bone at maturity will lose it in the same way as their less well-endowed cohorts, but in old age they can still be left with enough bone to bear the body weight and to resist the breaking forces of muscle action without developing fractures.

Some of the factors which can induce or worsen osteoporosis are:

*Immobilization* whether due to fracture, arthrodesis or ankylosis of a joint, or prolonged splinting. Probably, where the old are concerned, sitting or lying about for long periods is the most potent cause of generalized osteoporosis

*Excessive adrenal corticosteroid activity*, either from Cushing's disease or drug therapy with steroids

*Calcium deficiency.* The importance of calcium deficiency in osteoporosis has been hotly debated. On balance it seems likely that it plays an inconstant and minor role.

## The clinical features

Severe osteoporosis can exist for many years without causing any symptoms, but when these occur the spine is usually affected earliest and worst. *Backache*, the cardinal symptom, is usually felt in the lower dorsal or lumbar regions; it is relieved by lying flat and made worse by twisting movements of the trunk. Girdle pain from nerve root compression occurs rarely, though vague 'sciatica' pain is common. The symptoms are often curiously intermittent: sudden exacerbations of pain are followed by months of freedom, without any corresponding objective change.

*'Crush fractures'* of one or more dorsal or lumbar vertebrae are mundane in osteoporosis, though there is rarely any crescendo of pain to signal their occurrence.

The objective physical signs of osteoporosis are unimpressive: a dorsal kyphosis, without much scoliosis, and smoothly rounded unless angulated by the wedging effect of a crush fracture, is almost always present. Loss of height and downward inclination of the head are two by-products of severe crush fractures.

Osteoporosis also predisposes to fractures of other bones

than the vertebral bodies. The neck of the femur, pubic rami, forearm and upper end of the humerus can be involved.

*X-ray findings*

Loss of radiological density in the vertebral bodies is the main finding, though standardization of bone density is difficult. A 'crush fracture' gives rise to reduced height of the vertebral body affected and in the lateral view the vertebra is wedged, with the narrow end directed internally.

*Treatment*

Prophylaxis being better than treatment, it is important to *avoid immobilization* either of a limb or the whole person: the tendency of some old people not to stand when they can sit and not to sit when they can lie, needs to be resisted.

*Therapy with sex hormones* is generally held to be of value in arresting the progress of osteoporosis (bone, once lost, cannot be renewed). For women, an oestrogen such as dienoestrol 0·3 mg one to three times daily can be given in courses lasting one month with a gap of one week between. For men, testosterone, 25 to 50 mg, can be taken daily without break. The anabolic agents, beloved of muscle-men and allegedly non-virilizing in women, have not been conclusively shown to be superior to the sex hormones mentioned.

There is no evidence that calcium supplements to the diet are of benefit, though it is sensible to ensure that the intake is adequate. The same arguments apply to vitamin D: if there is doubt about the adequacy of the dietary intake—and there often is in old people—a daily supplement of 500 units of calciferol orally can safely be given.

## Osteomalacia

Osteomalacia is due to lack of calcium in the skeleton and is the adult equivalent of childhood rickets, the basic disturbance being lack of the physiological activity of vitamin D. This lack can be due to:

*Simple dietary deficiency.* The diet of a few old people is deficient in vitamin D: the illusion that 'best butter' is superior to margarine and the common prejudice against cheese because of its dreaded 'binding' effect are two contributory factors.

*Malabsorption.* Vitamin D is fat-soluble, so a deficiency is common in steatorrhoea or in the 'stagnant loop' syndrome.

*Inadequate skin exposure to sunlight,* the ultraviolet component of which is needed for vitamin D synthesis, is another factor. About 10 per cent of old people in the United Kingdom are housebound and only an eccentric minority of the remainder will ever expose large areas of their skin to the fickle sunlight of the British Isles.

*Previous partial gastrectomy* can cause vitamin D lack, usually after a lapse of several years.

*The clinical features*

Often, the diagnosis of osteomalacia is made simply by keeping the possibility in mind when the patient's circumstances (they are almost invariably women) pre-dispose to the disease.

Common symptoms and signs are:

> Generalized muscle pains, especially backache
> Muscular weakness and stiffness
> Tenderness of the bones to pressure
> Pathological fracture
> Skeletal deformity.

Generalized muscle pains are common but often excite little interest and are dismissed as 'rheumatic' or 'neurotic'. Examination will, however, often reveal striking muscle weakness; this is due to a specific myopathy, associated with changes in the electromyograph. The weakness affects the *proximal limb girdle muscles.* Flexors of the hip are worst affected and make it difficult to lift the foot clear of the ground: the difficulty is avoided by adopting a stumpy, waddling gait. In the shoulder, much more rarely involved, abduction and elevation of the arm are weak and interfere with dressing and hair toilet.

The bones are softened, as a result of the calcium deficiency, and this has three effects:

They are *painful on weight bearing*

They are *tender to pressure*—the ribs and sternum are most accessible for this sign and they *fracture easily.*

*Confirmation of the diagnosis*

On X-ray the bones are less dense than normal. Most often

affected are the vertebral bodies, the upper and lower surfaces of which become concave ('codfish vertebra'). Crush fractures are not typical of osteomalacia, but osteoporosis coexists frequently and then crush fractures are by no means rare.

One sign which is pathognomonic, though not always present, is '*Looser's zones*'. These resemble crack fractures, they are perpendicular to the external surface and reach to it, with denser ridges of apparent callus on either side. The ribs, scapula, neck of the humerus and femoral neck are common sites for the zones.

There are usually *serum biochemical abnormalities* in osteomalacia, in contrast with osteoporosis. The serum calcium concentration is low or normal and inorganic phosphorus is low. These two abnormalities are rapidly abolished by vitamin D treatment.

The serum alkaline phosphatase activity is raised, but this, on the other hand, responds to vitamin D only after several weeks or months.

Bone biopsy is not routinely necessary for making the diagnosis: histological examination of a section (without decalcification) will show the typical *osteoid bone formation*.

## Treatment

Treatment consists of giving calciferol (and removing whatever condition is predisposing to the vitamin D deficiency). Oral calciferol treatment is preferable, in a dose of 1000 to 5000 units daily, but if there is difficulty with oral therapy, or doubt whether it will be taken regularly, a depôt intramuscular injection of 50 000 units of vitamin D can be given. The serum calcium concentration often falls sharply once treatment is begun and oral calcium supplements (1 gram of calcium hydrogen phosphate daily) are needed during this period.

Vitamin D therapy is not entirely without risk. Excessive dosage can rapidly cause hypercalcaemia, with the attendant risk of calcifying soft tissues or organs. It is, therefore, wise to keep the patient under observation and to control calciferol dosage according to the serum calcium concentration. Very rarely, a patient will become addicted to vitamin D for its euphorizing effect.

## Paget's disease

Osteitis deformans is a patchy disease of the skeleton. In the affected area there is simultaneous resorption of bone and the formation of new bone, but the new bone has a disordered architectural pattern and is unsatisfactory in an engineering sense. It lacks the stress-resistence of normal bone and is more liable to fracture.

Any bone can be affected: the usual victims are the skull, pelvis, vertebral bodies, femur, clavicle and tibia, usually more than one bone is involved. Those bones affected are enlarged, thickened and, where accessible to touch, are warmer than normal due to the large blood flow. Deafness from involvement of the auditory ossicles is common and *bone pain* is usually the only complaint.

Two complications of Paget's disease are:

*High-output heart failure:* this occurs only with severe, wide-spread bone lesions and even then is rare

*Osteogenic sarcoma* is a more common and sinister complication of the disease.

### Treatment

A recent development is the treatment of Paget's disease with the hormone calcitonin. The dose is measured in biologically standardized 'M.R.C. units'—about 150 units daily, by intramuscular injection is a customary dose.

Prolonged treatment with human calcitonin is believed to improve the radiological pattern of bone modelling, but extended treatment is very expensive. Briefer periods of treatment, 2 or 3 weeks, often produce a remission of bone pain lasting up to one year.

Pig and salmon calcitonin are available but they tend to produce antibodies, and resistance to the biochemical action of the hormone can develop.

## Fractures

One fracture site towers in importance above all others in the elderly—the upper end of the femur. Women are affected three times more often than men and osteoporosis, again much commoner in the female sex, is a major pre-disposing factor.

Fracture of the femoral neck is always a major event, and often a catastrophe which transforms life for the worse in an old person: it has a substantial immediate death-rate and leaves a legacy in some of chronic invalidism. Within this general framework there are, however, two completely different types of femoral fracture, depending on the anatomical site (see Fig. 11.1).

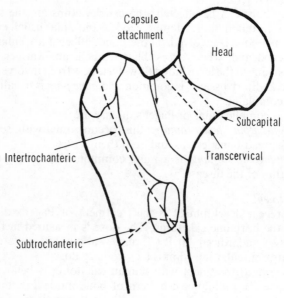

Fig. 11.1  Diagram of various types of fracture of the neck of the femur.

*Subcapital and transcervical fractures* (about 60 per cent of the total)

These occur within the hip joint capsule and have these abnormalities:

The immediate mortality is low.
The incidence of bony non-union is rather high, due to the precarious blood supply of the distal fragment: avascular necrosis leads to mushrooming and disintegration of the femoral head.
Because of non-union, convalescence is prolonged with

all the attendant evils of protracted immobilization, i.e. pressure sores, pneumonia, mental confusion and urinary incontinence.

*Intertrochanteric and subtrochanteric* (about 40 per cent of the total)

These are extra-capsular and have these special features:

The immediate mortality is substantial (for no very clear reason except that these patients tend to be older)

The prospects of bony union are good in those who survive the acute phase, since the fracture occurs through cancellous bone with a good blood supply

Since non-union is rare, convalescence is relatively quick and the long-term mortality and morbidity are lower.

*Causes*

Fractures in young people usually require severe direct trauma, but in old people they often occur without external violence. The vast majority are in fact due to falls occurring in the home. Direct impact of the fractured area against the ground is probably only one factor. Normally, the main breaking stress on bones comes from the powerful forces exerted by muscles inserted into them: body weight plays only a minor part. Old people have reduced postural sense and poor righting reflexes: they trip or stumble easily and recover clumsily, and incoordinate muscle contractions in attempts to recover balance probably have a part to play in femoral neck fractures.

About three-quarters of all femoral fractures occur in the home or near it, the commonest place being the dining or sitting room, followed by the kitchen and bedroom. Surprisingly, the bathroom or lavatory is an unusual venue for a fall.

Tripping or stumbling over flooring materials is by far the commonest single cause; a ruck in a carpet or a slippery mat are frequently responsible. Falls from a chair or bed, 'drop attacks' and giddiness are other common circumstances.

Falls outside the home occur on irregular pavements or backyards, and at the kerbside. Slippery surfaces, especially ice, are frequently inculpated and the farther north in the British Isles the larger the part ice plays.

In all these kinds of fall, poor illumination, poor vision, confusion and distraction play a consistent part. Femoral fracture is also a relatively common event in patients with hemiplegia; they fall to the side of the stroke and fracture that hip. The incidence of femoral fracture is also high in psycho-geriatric wards.

## Treatment

Reduction of the fracture followed by internal fixation of the fragments by means of a pin driven from the outside into the femoral head along the axis of the neck and secured in some types by a plate screwed into the shaft of the femur is the usual immediate treatment. There are many kinds of fixation devices and selection from them depends on the type of fracture and the orthopaedic surgeon's preference. In a small proportion of cases the femoral head is excised and a plastic prosthesis inserted as a first measure.

Technical manipulation of the fracture is, however, only one part of the treatment. The immediate postoperative care, with emphasis on the prevention of pressure sores, prompt treatment of pulmonary infections and avoidance of pulmonary embolism, is just as important if chronic invalidism is to be averted.

In a small minority, surgical measures are not undertaken because of the patient's poor general condition or some specific contraindication. If they survive, some of these patients get a useful false hip joint on which weight can be borne, though with difficulty. Failure to obtain satisfactory union most commonly occurs because of: (1) a poor blood supply to the distal fragment in a subcapital fracture—the head flattens and can disintegrate or be almost completely resorbed; (2) unsatisfactory internal fixation due to the pin either not being in the true axis of the neck and along a diameter of the femoral head, or being driven too far and protruding into the acetabular space—a painful situation which requires the pin to be removed.

Prophylactic treatment directed at removing or minimizing the environmental causes of falling mentioned above could probably do much to reduce the fractured femur incidence.

## Prognosis

The mortality of fractured femur rises sharply after the age of 70 and reaches 50 per cent at 90 years or more. Death is in the great majority due to pneumonia or pulmonary embolism.

FURTHER READING

Clark, A.N.G. (1968) Factors in fracture of the female femur: A clinical study of the environmental, physical, medical and preventative aspects of this injury. *Gerontologia Clinica*, **10**, 257–270.

# Part Three: Special Features of Disease in Old Age

# 12. Anaemia

Anaemia is not a single disease entity: it is an effect of many common diseases and for this reason is an important and common problem in geriatric medicine.

One widely used definition of 'anaemia' in old age is the World Health Organization criterion of a peripheral blood haemoglobin concentration below 13·0 g per 100 ml in men and below 12·0 g in women. Defined by this criterion alone, anaemia affects about 7 per cent of the elderly population living at home; the prevalence in geriatric wards is much higher—up to 40 per cent in some series.

Although virtually the whole gamut of diseases which cause anaemia in early adult life also occur in old age, the vast bulk of anaemias, both at home and in hospitals, can be accounted for by three kinds:

Iron deficiency

Megaloblastic anaemias

Anaemia associated with chronic diseases.

This chapter will concentrate on these three types.

*Effects of aging on the blood*

Not a great deal is known about the effects of aging on haemopoiesis. The pattern of development of red and white cells is not qualitatively changed as age advances, but the peripheral marrow contains substantially fewer haemopoietic cells and its capacity to respond to artificial stimuli, such as certain polysaccharides and corticosteroids, is reduced. The regenerative response to blood loss or to treatment of pernicious anaemia is also less brisk in old people.

The life-span of red cells is not changed as age advances and their morphology shows no important alteration.

*The symptoms and signs of anaemia in the elderly*

It has already been emphasized that anaemia is a symptom

and not a disease entity, hence the 'big three' listed above, iron lack, megaloblastosis and some chronic diseases, have many clinical features in common: their accurate separation leans very heavily on specialized haematological investigations.

Old people experience much the same symptoms of anaemia as do younger patients: easy fatigue, dyspnoea and palpitations on exertion, dizziness and anorexia are five common symptoms, but no single one nor any combination of them is diagnostic of anaemia. Other non-specific symptoms include headache, irritability, failure of concentration and coldness of limbs.

Where signs are concerned, *pallor* is the most useful. It can be detected in the face, palms of the hands and mucous membranes of the lips or conjunctivae: each of these sites can at times be misleading taken individually, but together they provide a reliable clinical guide to anaemia. Minor degrees of anaemia cannot be detected with certainty, but an experienced observer will rarely be in doubt that the haemoglobin level is less than 10 g per 100 ml.

Other signs which have value are:

> *Dystrophic nail changes.* Full-blown koilonychia is almost pathognomonic of iron deficiency, but lesser changes such as brittleness, flattening and ridging of the nails are common in the absence of anaemia and are of little diagnostic value.
>
> *Glossitis.* The tongue is reddened and sore, and smooth because the papillae are shrunken and flat. These changes occur in many patients with pernicious anaemia and in a few with iron deficiency.

Three other frequent signs of anaemia, whatever its origin, are:

Oedema of the ankles
Low grade fever, and
Weight loss.

There are also a few features of anaemia special to the elderly:

1. The anaemia is often very severe by the time the patient seeks advice: this is probably due mainly to misguided

acceptance of symptoms as one of the inevitable evils of getting old, in part to reluctance to bother the medical attendant, and in part to adjustments in the oxygen dissociation curve.

2. Congestive heart failure is a common presenting feature, no doubt because the patient often has intrinsic heart disease as well, and the stage is already set for the development of heart failure.

3. Mental symptoms are common and may dominate the scene. Here again, anaemia may be simply the final factor tipping the balance in a patient with failing mental powers.

## Iron deficiency anaemia

Iron deficiency is by far the commonest kind of anaemia in old people and is of special importance because it is often— much more so than in young patients—the presenting feature of some major disease.

The three basic mechanisms of iron deficiency are:
Blood loss
Malabsorption
Malnutrition.

### Iron balance

Iron deficiency anaemia arises when the amount of iron present and available in the marrow falls below that needed for haemoglobin synthesis in developing red cells. But this will only arise after the main body iron stores, chiefly in the liver have already been heavily drained. These reserves are large, about 1000 mg, and are kept constant through a sensitive feed-back mechanism in intestinal epithelial cells, which adjusts the amount of iron absorbed from the diet to the amount lost from within.

The daily iron loss is only about 1 mg in health, chiefly as exfoliated intestinal cells, plus a small leakage of blood. The internal economy of iron is astonishingly efficient; about 20 mg of iron pass into the plasma each day from lysed red cells, but this is re-cycled to the marrow and re-used with very little waste. However, with a normal iron intake, there is only a small margin available for adjusting to increased losses. The dietary iron of old people in the UK ranges from 8 to 12 mg per day, but only about 3 to 5 mg of this can be absorbed even when absorption is stretched to full capacity. If blood loss exceeds 15 ml per day (7 mg of elemental iron) then even if absorption be increased to the maximum possible, the current iron account will start to be over-drawn and to be replenished from the body stores of iron.

*The peripheral blood in iron deficiency anaemia*

The typical changes in iron deficiency anaemia, in addition to the obvious reduction of haemoglobin concentration, are as follows:

1. The mean corpuscular volume ('MCV') is reduced, often to the range 65 to 70 cubic μm.

2. The mean total corpuscular haemoglobin ('MCH') is consistently reduced below 30 picograms. Much more importance is now attached to the total haemoglobin content of the 'average' red cell (MCH) than to the MCHC, when automatic counting methods are used.

3. The blood film reveals red cells smaller than normal on average (in keeping with the low 'MCV'), but there is a wide range of sizes (anisocytosis) and of shapes (poikilocytosis). The colour density of the red cells is reduced, presumably due to proportionate thinning of the red cells as part of a general reduction in their size. Two unusual cells, 'pencil' cells, so called because of their long elliptical shape, and 'target' cells, which have a central very pale portion, are typical of iron deficiency anaemia.

4. The platelets are often increased, and in severe degrees of anaemia can reach values of 0·5 to 1 million per mm³.

5. The white cells show no characteristic change.

The further investigation of a patient found to have these haematological changes involves three aspects:

Proof that there is in fact iron deficiency

Detection of possible causes of blood loss

Detection of malabsorption or inadequate iron intake.

Proof of iron deficiency can be obtained by measurement of the *serum iron concentration* and the *total iron binding capacity of the serum* (TIBC). A third commonly used piece of information is the 'percentage iron binding' which is derived from these two measurements. In straightforward iron deficiency anaemia, the findings will be:

A reduction of the serum iron concentration below 12$\mu$ moles per litre (60 $\mu$g per ml)

High normal or increased serum TIBC

Reduction of 'percentage saturation' to 16 per cent or less.

Sometimes the TIBC is low normal or reduced (especially if there is present another general disease associated with low protein synthesis), and then the percentage saturation can be normal. In these circumstances the court of appeal will be staining of a marrow section for haemosiderin; its complete absence in the presence of equivocal serum iron findings, will usually settle the matter in favour of iron deficiency.

The second aspect, detection of blood loss, is of major practical importance. No anaemia of any type in old people should be handled without the question 'is underlying blood loss an element in the anaemia?' being considered.

The first requirements for answering this question are:

1. A detailed enquiry into the patient's symptoms, with special reference to the possible sources of bleeding
2. A complete physical examination.

Many old people will not readily volunteer facts about their medical history: they will wait to be asked about them. The old are also naturally more reluctant, simply from modesty, about 'intimate' symptoms such as rectal or vaginal bleeding or discharge. It is therefore worth asking *direct* questions about:

1. Known previous anaemia?
2. Previous admissions to hospital and any surgical procedures undergone (especially partial gastrectomy)?
3. Recent changes in bowel habit: constipation, diarrhoea or alternation of these?
4. Rectal or vaginal bleeding or discharge?
5. Has haematuria occurred?
6. Special dietary habits (vegetarianism, slimming, diabetic) and food prejudices?
7. What drugs are being taken? This question should include 'over the counter' purchases of aspirin, Alka-Seltzer, etc. as well as any enquiry into treatment with corticosteroids and the antirheumatic drugs.

*Physical examination*

Special attention should be paid to the abdomen, the anus should be inspected and a manual rectal and vaginal examination done. If there is a history of rectal bleeding or discharge, sigmoidoscopy should be performed after full preparation. A thorough clinical examination of this kind may well give some positive hint of the underlying disease, but it will often be negative; the question then will be—'how far am I justified in pursuing special examinations in order to exclude an underlying early bowel neoplasm?' and to this question there is no stereotyped answer. In old people who have severe physical or mental disabilities such as a total hemiplegia or advanced dementia, where the prognosis is already limited and the quality of life inevitably poor, it is often justifiable to spare the patient the discomfort of radiological examinations of the bowel when the level of suspicion is low, though the wishes of the patient and the patient's relatives must obviously be taken into account here.

If it is decided to go further with investigation the next logical step is to examine the stools for 'occult blood', and persistently positive occult blood tests give strong encouragement for radiological examination of the bowel.

*The treatment of iron deficiency anaemia*

The treatment consists, in the great majority of patients, of giving iron-containing drugs by mouth: only rarely is it necessary to resort to intramuscular or intravenous therapy, but therapeutic preferences vary and some physicians may prefer the rapidity and certainty of parenteral therapy.

The daily oral dosage is 100 to 150 mg of elemental iron, whether the anaemia be mild or severe.

Three widely used British Pharmacopoeial preparations are:

Ferrous Sulphate Tablet B.P. (200 mg) dose 1 b.d.

Ferrous Fumarate Tablet B.P. dose 1 b.d.

Ferrous Gluconate Tablet B.P. dose 1 b.d.


Failure to obtain the expected response to oral iron occurs when:

The drug therapy is not being properly taken

The amount of iron prescribed is inadequate

Blood loss continues to outstrip new haemoglobin synthesis.

Some other disease has developed during treatment, or the original diagnosis was wrong.

There is more severe malabsorption than has been recognized.

*Iron deficiency due to malabsorption*

The main causes are:

1. Chronic atrophic gastritis
2. Partial or total gastrectomy
3. Small intestine resection
4. Steatorrhoea: idiopathic
    pancreatic
    drug induced (neomycin)
5. Chronic diarrhoea with 'intestinal hurry':
    regional ileitis
    gastro-colic fistula
    drug induced

The relation between chronic atrophic gastritis and iron deficiency is a longstanding and continuing debate. It now seems likely that (1) primary chronic atrophic gastritis can cause iron deficiency, probably not so much through a failure of iron absorption as from increased faecal iron loss from the larger number of parietal cells shed daily, though if gastric function is impaired to the point of achlorhydria this will also impede absorption, and (2) iron deficiency can cause atrophic gastritis.

*Gastric or ileojejunal resection*

Many patients who have undergone extensive resection of the stomach or small intestine will ultimately get severe iron deficiency: it can be prevented by prophylactic iron therapy. The history and abdominal scar make diagnosis easy.

*Steatorrhoea*

The diagnosis of excessive fat loss in the stool can often be made by inspection of the stools: they are bulky, pale, foul-smelling and will float in water. A 24-hour collection of stools will contain more than 4 g of fat but several successive days' stools need to be examined because steatorrhoea is often intermittent. The xylose tolerance test will usually indicate impaired absorption and if further confirmation is needed a jejunal biopsy by the Crosby capsule will often reveal mucosal atrophy.

## Megaloblastic anaemias

Megaloblastic anaemia is, by definition, an anaemia characterized by the presence in the marrow of large nucleated red cell precursors which do not occur in the normal sequence of erythrocyte development. The peripheral blood is 'macrocytic', i.e. the red cells are larger than usual, but this term and 'megaloblastic' are not synonymous: all megaloblastic anaemias give a macrocytic blood picture, but not all the diseases causing macrocytosis are of megaloblastic nature.

For practical purposes megaloblastic anaemia in the elderly is due to either vitamin $B_{12}$ or 'folate' deficiency. The $B_{12}$ deficiency is almost always due to *pernicious anaemia*, a disease caused primarily by exhaustion of the ability of gastric parietal cells to produce a transport protein, the 'intrinsic factor'. Deficiency of $B_{12}$ is only rarely of strictly nutritional origin. Folate deficiency, on the other hand, most often results from malnutrition, with malabsorption as a common factor.

*Folic acid* is so named because it occurs in the foliage of plants. As strictly defined chemically, folic acid occurs in nature in only small quantities, but partly or wholly hydrogenated derivatives of it, conjugated with one or more molecules of glutamic acid, have important biochemical functions, and it is these physiologically important derivatives which are now commonly lumped together under the term 'folate'. Human cells cannot synthesize folate from scratch, and are entirely dependent on dietary sources.

Folate taken in with the diet is absorbed and metabolized in the upper small intestine: it emerges from the epithelial cells into the blood stream as the 'transport form', 5-methyl tetrahydrofolic acid (THF). This can penetrate cells which, according to their biochemical function, transform it into other derivatives of THF destined to take part in the metabolism of certain amino-acids, in the *de novo* synthesis of purines, in the initiation of peptide chain synthesis and—a function probably of special importance in the context of megaloblastic anaemia—in the biosynthesis of a deoxyri-bonucleotide containing thymidine, one of the characteristic bases of the nucleic acids.

*Vitamin B$_{12}$* cannot be synthesized by plants or man, but is widely made by bacteria. After ingestion it is stored in many animal tissues, and human beings depend for supply on their carnivorous habits and on bacterial contamination of food. The daily requirement is very small, only about 2 μg per day.

Vitamin B$_{12}$ is transported through the stomach and upper small intestine as a complex with 'intrinsic factor', a glyco-protein produced by the parietal cells of the stomach, usually in considerable excess. Without the protection given by this complex, vitamin B$_{12}$ is destroyed by pepsin in the stomach. After absorption in the lower small intestine vitamin B$_{12}$ is transported in plasma by carrier proteins called transcobala-mins. The liver usually contains about 1.5 mg, enough to meet requirements for about 2 years.

By far the commonest cause of megaloblastic anaemia in the old is pernicious anaemia. A deficiency of folate is also well established as a cause, but there is some disagreement about its prevalence. In the population at large, 'pure' folate defi-ciency causing severe anaemia is much less common than pernicious anaemia, but in hospital series the two are about

Table 12.1 Causes of folate deficiency

---

*Inadequate intake*
  Immobility, social isolation, apathy, poverty
*Malabsorption*
  Gluten-sensitive enteropathy, dermatitis herpetiformis, small bowel resection, chronic pancreatitis
*Increased use*
  Neoplasms and reticuloses with rapid, primitive cell production
*Inhibition of activity*
  Drugs. Dihydrofolate reductase inhibitors. Methotrexate: trimethoprim (very rare, prolonged use only), diphenylhydantoin (prolonged use as anticonvulsant)
*Excessive loss*
  Skin diseases with rapid cell turnover (psoriasis, exfoliative dermatitis) Liver damage, chronic biliary disease

---

equally common. Minor degrees of folate deficiency, not clinically expressed as anaemia are common, however, since there is a host of conditions which can cause folate lack (see Table 12.1).

It is important to remember that pernicious anaemia and nutritional folate deficiency commonly occur together. Sometimes, iron deficiency too, in the old.

*Clinical findings in megaloblastic anaemia*

The general features of any severe anaemia have already been described. The specific features of pernicious anaemia are glossitis and the occasional development of subacute combined degeneration of the spinal cord; the common symptoms are weakness and ataxia of the legs and a complaint of symmetrical paraesthesiae, often of a bizarre kind.

Occasionally, a patient with megaloblastic anaemia will prove to have carcinoma of the stomach. Suspicion of this will be aroused by unusually severe anorexia, bloating after meals, weight loss or vomiting. Mere suspicion is sufficient justification for barium meal studies, as the appearance of an abdominal mass or glands in the posterior triangle of the neck is an indication of advanced and usually inoperable disease.

The symptoms of folate deficiency are those of anaemia *per se* and of the underlying gastrointestinal disease when malabsorption is the cause. When folate deficiency is severe and of purely nutritional origin, multiple water-soluble vitamin deficiencies will probably coexist, though flagrant clinical signs of lack of riboflavin, pyridoxine, nicotinic acid or ascorbic acid are very rare.

*The peripheral blood in megaloblastic anaemia*

Typical findings in an uncomplicated case are:

*The mean corpuscular volume* (MCV) is *increased*—in pernicious anaemia often as high as 120 to 130 $\mu^3$. In folic acid deficiency it is usually in the range 96 to 110 $\mu^3$ The normal range is 76 to 96 $\mu^3$.

*The mean corpuscular haemoglobin concentration* (MCHC) is normal.

*The mean corpuscular haemoglobin is increased* in proportion with the rise of MCV. The normal range is 27 to 32 pg.

*The peripheral blood film* shows large red cells of normal or dense colour and often polychromatic (blue colour is due to persistence of cytoplasmic RNA). The cells are more variable than normal in both size and shape; pear-shaped red cells are common. In severe anaemia a few nuclear ghosts or 'Howell-Jolly bodies' are present.

*The white cell count* (normal range 4000 to 11 000 per mm$^3$) is usually reduced, often to the range 2000 to 3000 per mm$^3$. There is an absolute fall of polymorphs, but those present are often 'hypersegmented'; there are cells with six lobes and 10 per cent or more will have five lobes.

*The platelet count* is either normal or reduced: it can be very low and then has sinister prognostic value.

*The serum iron concentration* is *high* (above 180 μg per 100 ml) and the total iron binding capacity is usually normal, hence the percentage saturation is also high.

If all these features are present in the peripheral blood, a provisional diagnosis of megaloblastic anaemia can be made, but proof positive needs a haematologist's examination of the bone marrow, which will show hypercellularity, the characteristic megaloblasts (their number runs parallel with the severity of anaemia) and profuse reticulo-endothelial iron.

When anaemia is very slight both the peripheral blood and marrow findings can be equivocal. In these circumstances a therapeutic trial of vitamin B$_{12}$ or folate will probably give a more satisfactory answer than the biochemical tests available (formiminoglutamic acid (FIGLU) excretion in urine after histidine loading for folate, and methylmalonate excretion in urine after valine loading for vitamin B$_{12}$): these tests require an overnight fast and accurate urine collection, neither of which manoeuvres is really feasible with the very old.

Having established that the anaemia is in fact megaloblastic, it remains to be settled whether it is a pure deficiency of vitamin B$_{12}$, of folate or a mixed deficiency. Three measurements—serum vitamin B$_{12}$ concentration and the folate concentration of serum and red cells will settle the matter: the typical findings are tabulated overleaf.

| Deficiency | Serum vit-amin $B_{12}$ | Serum folate | Red cell folate |
| --- | --- | --- | --- |
| Vitamin $B_{12}$ deficiency | Low | Normal or high | Low |
| Folic acid lack | Normal | Low or very low | Low |
| Vitamin $B_{12}$ and folate lack | Low | Low | Very low |

*Megaloblastic anaemia with iron deficiency*

In this case the MCV will not be so elevated, the peripheral blood film may show a 'double population' of microcytic and macrocytic cells, the serum iron concentration will not be raised, the percentage saturation of transferrin will not be so high, and the marrow will show little or no stainable iron and megaloblastic changes are inconspicuous.

## The treatment of megaloblastic anaemias

*Pernicious anaemia*

The treatment consists in essence of intramuscular injections of vitamin $B_{12}$, given for the rest of the patient's life (a fact which needs to be clearly explained to both the patient and his relatives).

The preferred drug is hydroxycyanocobalamin ('Neocytamen') given in doses of 1000 $\mu$g at weekly intervals for the first four to six weeks. Maintenance therapy consists of injections of 250 $\mu$g at about monthly intervals. If laboratory facilities are plentiful the response to treatment can be maintained by measuring the reticulocyte count daily; the peak at five to seven days will reach 40 per cent of the red cells with an initial count of 1·0 million per $mm^3$.

It is wise to keep patients under supervision for the first three months of therapy. Failure to sustain the response to therapy can be due to these factors:

1. The injections are not being given, or not in adequate amounts

2. Iron deficiency has developed: the serum iron concentration will then be low. Oral iron therapy will usually put this right

3. The diagnosis is wrong and the possibility of an underlying gastric neoplasm should be considered

4. There is folate deficiency, though this will usually have been detected at the initial investigation, in which case folic acid 5 mg t.d.s. will have been given from the beginning.

*Note: Do not give folic acid alone before giving vitamin $B_{12}$ therapy to pernicious anaemia patients:* subacute combined degeneration of the cord can be worsened or precipitated.

## Treatment of folic acid deficiency anaemia

The treatment consists of: (1) giving folic acid by mouth and (2) detecting and treating any malabsorption state that exists. The dose of folic acid is by 5 mg tablets three or four times daily. Where oral therapy is not practicable, folic acid can be given by intramuscular injection, 15 mg in 1 ml once daily. If it is a purely nutritional deficiency of folate, then other vitamins are also likely to be lacking and should be replaced by a multivitamin preparation (Tab. vitamin B Co. Forte B.P.C.). Replacement of body folate stores normally occurs within a few days, but if the factors causing folate deficiency are likely to recur, prophylactic treatment is continued.

Iron deficiency can develop in folate deficiency just as in pernicious anaemia.

## Anaemia of chronic disease

### Chronic infections

Anaemia is often associated with common chronic infections in old age: chronic pyelocystitis, infected leg ulcers, indolent soft tissue infections, infected pressure sores, diverticulitis, tuberculosis and many others less common.

Only severe infections and those of long standing will cause anaemia, and even then the disorder is usually mild. The basic causes are several, complex and ill-understood, but the three main mechanisms are disturbed iron metabolism, impaired haemoglobin synthesis and depression of marrow function.

The infective process has an intrinsic action on iron metabolism: the plasma iron concentration is low and (in contrast with iron deficiency anaemia) the plasma total iron-binding capacity is also low, hence the percentage iron saturation is normal. Iron excretion is not increased and the body stores of iron remain normal or increased; in the marrow there is abundant haemosiderin, but sideroblasts are reduced.

The red cells are normocytic and normochromic as a rule, but in severe anaemia they can be microcytic and hypochromic.

The anaemia of chronic infection does not respond to oral iron therapy and is best treated symptomatically by repeated small transfusions of packed red cells. However, the most important aspect is to detect and eradicate the underlying infection.

## Uraemia (chronic renal failure)

Anaemia is common in chronic renal failure. It is rarely severe unless the blood urea persistently exceeds 100 mg per 100 ml but beyond this range the depression of haemoglobin is well correlated with the glomerular filtration rate. Recurrent pyelo-cystitis, polycystic kidneys and diabetic nephropathy are three common causes of structural renal disease, but long-standing pre- and postrenal uraemia will also cause anaemia.

As with chronic infections, the main causes of this anaemia are several and not well understood. Erythropoiesis is depressed, probably due to the uraemic environment rather than to lack of erythropoetin. Iron metabolism is also disturbed but the findings are erratic and often difficult to interpret. The serum iron is low and plasma iron turnover is reduced, though an unusually large part of the turnover enters tissue reticulendothelial cells. Red cell survival is shortened.

## Rheumatoid arthritis

Rheumatoid arthritis is common in the elderly and is often accompanied by anaemia. Two types of blood disturbance are recognized: the commoner has a normocytic but hypochromic picture in the peripheral blood; the rarer is a megaloblastic anaemia due to folate deficiency. The normocytic anaemia usually signifies active rheumatoid arthritis and is associated with a high sedimentation rate. It is worth remembering that a great many of these patients are already taking large doses of aspirin or other antirheumatic drugs; these are a potent source of quiet intestinal bleeding, and can easily complicate the blood picture.

*Treatment*

The anaemia does not usually respond to iron therapy, but the haemoglobin usually rises after parenteral iron therapy. Steroid therapy corrects the iron abnormalities and this seems to be the optimum treatment, provided there are no other factors in the patient's general condition which contraindicate it.

The megaloblastic anaemia of rheumatoid arthritis is due to folate deficiency and has the generic biochemical and haematological features of this condition (see p. 126).

FURTHER READING

D.H.S.S. (1972) *A Nutrition Survey of the Elderly.* H.M.S.O.

Israels, M.C.G. & Delamore, I.W. (Eds) (1972) Haematological aspects of systemic disease. In *Clinics in Haematology* **1,** No. 3, October.

Thomas J.H. & Powell, D.E.B. (1971) *Blood Disorders in the Elderly.* Bristol: John Wright & Sons.

# 13. Heart Disease

Heart disease accounts for about one-third of deaths, and for a vast amount of morbidity and disablement in old age. The dominant cause is ischaemia, closely followed by hypertension and, in third place, mixed cases where both these diseases are present. One or more episodes of congestive heart failure are common during the terminal phase of these diseases and auricular fibrillation is very prevalent.

Valvular heart disease constitutes only a minority of cardiac illnesses in old age and pulmonary heart disease is a rarity over 75, because the underlying chest disease has usually run its course by then.

*Physiopathological changes in the heart in old people*

The aorta loses elasticity as age advances. For a given stroke volume this demands a rise of the pulse pressure, which is achieved by a rise of systolic pressure, but no material change in the diastolic.

There is, however, no important increase of cardiac work as a result of the increased pulse pressure.

'Brown atrophy', the classical description of changes in the aged myocardium, is characterized by a loss of heart weight and infiltration of the muscle cells by the pigment lipofuscin (cf. the changes in the brain in dementia), but it is doubtful whether these have any baleful functional significance.

The aging myocardium is certainly capable of hypertrophy in response to increased work and can also be 'trained' in the athletic sense. But both at rest and on exercize, old people achieve a given tissue oxygen uptake by adopting a lower cardiac output and higher (A-V) oxygen difference than younger people, so there is some natural mechanism conserving the work of the heart in old age.

Probably of more importance than these age-conditioned

changes in the aorta and myocardium is involvement of coronary vessels in the ubiquitous sclerotic lesions of medium sized arteries. For the last quarter of a century attention has been diverted from the earlier belief that these changes are 'degenerative' lesions, to investigation of the possibility that arteriosclerosis is primarily or mainly a metabolic disease, in which first the intima then the deeper layer of arteries, are infiltrated by lipids derived from the circulation. But the intimal, elastic and all layers of arteries are not only structurally but functionally inseparable, and evidence accumulates steadily to show that arteriosclerosis could be primarily a 'disease' of elastic tissue. On this hypothesis, mechanical fragmentation of the elastic laminae by the many millions of cardiac pulsations which distend arteries during lifetime, probably forms a framework for the systematic deposition of lipids.

## Clinical features

In virtually all aspects, bar the pattern of causation, heart disease is no different in old age from in youth. Many excellent reference works are available on heart disease in general, so this chapter deals only with some special features and 'problems' of heart disease in old age.

Two potentially misleading cardiovascular physical signs in old people are: unilateral obstruction of the jugular vein and the 'kinked carotid syndrome'.

Unilateral obstruction of the left jugular vein arises from compression of the left innominate vein between a tortuous aorta and the back of the manubrium sterni. Two observations will avoid a mistaken diagnosis of congestive heart failure: the pressure in the right jugular vein is normal, and the elevated venous pressure on the left side will fall to normal if the patient makes a maximal inspiration (the veins normally empty during inspiration).

The 'kinked carotid' presents as a powerful arterial pulsation just above the clavicle on the right-hand side. It occurs in short-necked elderly women, usually with systolic hypertension and a dilated aorta (it is rare in men), and can be mistaken for a carotid aneurysm.

## Systolic murmurs

A systolic murmur is a common physical finding in an old person and can present real difficulty to the student. Three questions will be in the mind: 'Is the murmur of organic origin or not?'; 'Does it originate in the aortic or the mitral valve or (very much rarer), in the other two heart valves?' and, 'Is it a benign murmur, i.e. unlikely to harm the patient?'

Other things being equal, the louder the murmur the more likely it is to be 'organic'. Murmurs which are well heard at the back of the chest, and any systolic murmur accompanied by a palpable thrill can be assumed to be of organic origin.

To decide whether a murmur originates in the aortic valve or in the mitral valve is a frequent source of difficulty. The signs which help to decide this are: the character of the noise, its position in the cardiac cycle; its evolution (i.e. 'diminuendo', 'crescendo' or 'level') and its selective distribution over the chest wall.

The character of the murmur is probably most decisive, but presents difficulties of communication: a group of people hearing the same noise and given a choice of adjectives will describe it with conflicting results: the exact meaning of the descriptive terms used can only be learnt by example. *Aortic* murmurs are almost always 'harsh or 'rough' but some have a musical, 'cooing' or 'mewing' element. *Mitral* murmurs are 'blowing' or 'soft' (this last term is often ambiguously used to mean 'quiet'. *Innocent* murmurs (i.e. not of organic origin) are as a rule blowing in character, but some are 'superficial' or 'scratchy'; in contrast with organic murmurs, they often vary much with respiration.

### The distribution of the noise

Aortic murmurs are usually loudest in the second right interspace but, in addition, are often widely heard over the whole chest wall and not so rarely are actually maximal in the apical region. Mitral murmurs, on the other hand, are much less likely to be widely distributed or to be heard best at the 'base of the heart' (i.e. the second interspaces near the sternum); they are typically maximal in the apical region and radiate to the axilla. When doubt arises a useful rule is that a murmur which is very widely heard over the chest wall is more likely to be aortic than mitral (assuming it is one or the other) even if it is maximally heard in the mitral region. The harsh character of such a widely distributed murmur will give the game away.

'Innocent' murmurs are usually best heard in the second left interspace or left parasternal regions.

*The position in the cardiac cycle*

Aortic murmurs are *mid-systolic in timing and crescendo* in evolution. However, the gap between the first heart sound and onset of the murmur is always short and often not detectable clinically. When aortic stenosis is severe and the aortic second sound is absent or reduced, the murmur sounds like a short, isolated grunt.

Mitral murmurs, on the other hand, are *pansystolic* and more or less 'level' in loudness throughout.

'Innocent' murmurs are usually *late in systole:* there is a long, easily perceptible pause between the first cardiac sound and the beginning of the murmur.

Making the distinction between aortic *stenosis* and aortic *sclerosis* is a frequent dilemma. 'Stenosis' means there is increased cardiac work because of obstruction to outflow and so there is left ventricular hypertrophy, with its sinister prognostic implication. 'Sclerosis' means that the valve cusps are slightly rigid and thickened but offer no obstruction to outflow: it is a benign condition.

Both diseases cause an 'ejection' type of aortic systolic murmur. But the aortic element of the second sound is likely to be inaudible or reduced in intensity in stenosis, whereas it is normal in sclerosis. Most important of all, aortic sclerosis will show neither clinical nor electrocardiographic evidence of left ventricular hypertrophy.

## Symptoms and presentation of myocardial infarction in the elderly

Though complete absence of chest pain is very rare in acute myocardial infarction up to middle age, it is a mundane occurrence in old people. Only about one third of elderly patients present with the classical prolonged bout of substernal pain. Another third have atypical presentations such as:

1. The development of an acute confusional state
2. The abrupt appearance of severe dyspnoea
3. Persistent severe hypotension
4. Arterial embolism from clot formed over the infarction: the embolus may pass to the brain causing hemiplegia, or to non-cerebral arteries
5. Vomiting and weakness.

Finally, some myocardial infarcts in the aged are completely 'silent' and are discovered only in the electro-cardiograph. Perhaps this 'silent' presentation is due to the prevalence of chronic confusional states, especially in very old people: pain may be felt, but the patient is not articulate enough to identify it or complain of it, or may have forgotten the pain. The electrocardiograph is not intrinsically altered by old age, and any deviations from the normal have exactly the same significance as in the young.

## Orthostatic hypotension

A large fall of blood pressure on standing up is a common disability in old people and one which can often be rectified. It often presents as 'falling attacks' or as dizziness and weakness on standing, and postural hypotension should be considered in any old person who 'goes off his legs'. The symptoms are induced by sudden change to the erect posture and are worse in a hot environment and after a hot bath or a large meal. Occasionally a severe orthostatic fall of blood pressure occurs during micturition.

If the condition is once suspected, confirmation of the diagnosis is a simple matter, in gross cases by palpation of the radial pulse, which will become imperceptible when the patient stands up, or by measurement of the blood pressure in both the lying and standing position. The normal response to assuming the erect posture is first a brief dip of both the systolic and the diastolic pressures: the stabilized response is a slight rise of diastolic pressure with no material change in systolic: the resultant drop in pulse pressure is accompanied by a rise of pulse rate. If a measurement of blood pressure is to be made it is worth standardizing the technique: the patient first lies supine for 5 to 15 minutes, at the end of which the blood pressure is measured. The sphygmomanometer cuff is left on and the patient stands without holding himself rigid, and unsupported, if at all possible, for a timed two minutes (some patients cannot tolerate the procedure). The blood pressure is recorded again at the end of this time.

The majority of old people show the same response as the young on standing, but massive falls, associated with complaints of dizziness and fear of falling may occur. A systolic fall of 20 mm Hg or more is often arbitrarily taken as significant, but more important than the actual figure is whether there are associated symptoms.

The *causes* of postural hypotension are:

1. Drugs (a) Some antihypertensive drugs
   ganglion blocking agents (now rarely used)
   methyldopa
   reserpine
   (b) Unwanted effects of drugs affecting the nervous systems
   Laevodopa
   anticholinergic drugs
   tricyclic antidepressants
   phenothiazines
   barbiturates

2. An intrinsic degeneration of the autonomic elements concerned in blood pressure regulation. This can be idiopathic, or a complication of some neurological diseases which cause autonomic neuropathy—diabetes, tabes dorsalis or cerebellar degeneration.

3. A variety of bacterial and viral infections

4. Low cardiac output in ischaemic heart disease

5. Reduced blood volume in sodium depletion and haemorrhage

6. Commonest of all is a combination of these factors.

Drugs are probably the most common cause of postural hypotension in old people, and it is essential to find out what medication an affected patient is currently taking, and what discontinued prescriptions he could still be taking at his own indiscretion. The sensible course is to withdraw all but the essential drugs (usually none are) and observe the effect on blood pressure.

Treatment consists of removing any obvious cause, support of the venous return in the form of elastic stockings, and a graded programme of standing upright. If these measures alone are not enough, fludrocortisone, in a dose of 0·1 mg thrice daily will often help considerably, but this drug brings with it the problem of fluid retention.

## Hypertension in the elderly—to treat or not to treat?

When large groups of patients are studied, both the systolic and diastolic blood pressure continue to rise throughout adult life until the age of 65, after which there is no further increase. About 5 per cent of both men and women of 65 or over will have a systolic blood pressure exceeding 200 mm and a diastolic of 110 mm Hg or more. Blood pressure values of this kind are compatible with normal health and are, in themselves, no indication to give antihypertensive therapy. But each patient merits individual consideration, and the finding of associated gross left ventricular hypertrophy, dyspnoea on exertion, or paroxysms of dyspnoea while lying flat, or objective signs of left ventricular failure, would be good reasons to consider a modest reduction of the pressure.

A second problem is met in the occasional patient with much more severe pressure rises: for example, a sustained diastolic pressure of 130 to 140 mm Hg. It is the exception in old age for such patients to show the retinal and renal lesions of 'malignant hypertensiion' and most are simply severe instances of essential hypertension. While symptoms may be absent or even trivial when the hypertension is first discovered, the risk of developing heart failure or cerebral haemorrhage certainly exists at such pressure levels and antihypertensive therapy to prevent these is then well worth consideration.

Current geriatric opinion is, however, in general highly antagonistic to antihypertensive therapy in the old, largely because of the possible ill-effects of treatment, the worst of which are cerebral thrombosis or the induction of heart failure. Some at least of this attitude has doubtless been carried over from the early days of antihypertensive therapy with non-selective ganglion-blocking agents, when swingeing excessive falls of blood pressure with very low coronary or cerebral blood flow were often impossible to avoid.

Certainly there is good evidence that control of blood pressure does not benefit those patients who have already suffered a stroke. But there is very little information on the important problem of whether treating hypertension in non-hemiplegic elderly patients might reduce the incidence of later stroke—an event which carries a heavy and prolonged penalty for both the patients and their relatives.

Clearly, elderly patients require a specially cautious approach to antihypertensive therapy and only modest falls of pressure should be aimed at, with particular care to avoid severe postural or exertional pressure drops. This can usually be achieved by the use of a long-acting thiazide diuretic (with due care to avoid potassium deficiency) or by the use of methyldopa in doses of 250 to 500 mg daily.

## The special liability of old people to digitalis intoxication

Digitalis intoxication is common in old people. Doubtless this is mainly because heart failure is so common in old age and digitalis is very widely used to treat it. However, other factors are concerned in the prevalence of intoxication from this drug. First, digitalis is, unfortunately, often prescribed in standard quanta irrespective of age. In old people the lean body mass, on which digitalis is absorbed, is reduced, and myocardial concentrations of digitalis tend therefore to be high. Second, digitalis is excreted only by the kidneys, whose function is often reduced in old age, with a corresponding risk of drug accumulation. A digoxin dose of 0·25 mg twice daily could be well tolerated by a 25-year-old man of 100 kg body weight with normal renal function, but could cause serious toxicity in an 80-year-old woman weighing 40 kg with poor renal function.

Recent developments in immunological methods of assaying the digitalis group of drugs have defined levels above which toxicity is likely to appear (at about 2 ng per ml in the case of digoxin), but the between-individual variation is large and the methods are not routinely available. The detection of toxicity will continue to depend on clinical observation: the warning symptoms are nausea, a pulse rate below 60, bigeminy, frequent multifocal extrasystoles on the ECG, or the development of an abnormal cardiac rhythm. Special surveillance is necessary in patients made susceptible to potassium deficiency by the use of the thiazide diuretic.

In spite of its wide use for two centuries, the benefits to the failing heart from digitalis (other than its undoubted effect in slowing the ventricular response to the fibrillating atrium) are hard to demonstrate and are emphatically denied by some. On the other hand, the toxic effects are undeniable, are serious and can be fatal. It seems only provident, therefore, to err on the side of low rather than high dosage in digitalis therapy: the maximum potential benefit is less than the maximum possible harm. Where digoxin is concerned, doses as low as 0·0625 mg on alternate days can be enough for some patients, yet doses as high as 0·25 mg twice daily are often prescribed for a month or more. Such high doses are only exceptionally necessary and will eventually cause serious toxicity in many little old women with heart disease.

FURTHER READING

Caird, F.I., & Dall, J.L.C. (1973) The cardiovascular system. In *Textbook of Geriatric Medicine and Gerontology*, ed. Brocklehurst, J.C. Churchill Livingstone: Edinburgh.

# 14. Alimentary Disorders

## Upper alimentary tract

### Mouth and tongue

The tongue has long been regarded as a simple barometer of health and disease and nowhere is this more evident than in old age. It should always, therefore, be examined with care. Almost any systemic illness or illness of the alimentary tract will cause a white or brown furred tongue, a finding which of course is entirely non-specific. This must be distinguished from *oral moniliasis* (Candida infection or thrush) characterized by white patches not only on the tongue but also on the cheeks, gums and fauces. Monilial patches are not always easily removable (as food particles are) and the diagnosis can be confirmed by microscopic examination. Oral candidiasis is a common condition in the elderly and is easily treated with nystatin tablets, allowed to dissolve in the mouth, three times a day. Smoking, whether pipes or cigarettes, and ill-fitting dentures may also produce tongue changes with a white and sodden appearance of filiform papillae. In some cases there is a relationship between the white sodden filiform papillae and low levels of *nicotinic acid*. If no other cause is found for this appearance of the tongue, then it is worth prescribing B vitamins. Nicotinic acid deficiency may also produce a red and angry looking tongue. Vitamin $B_{12}$, folate and iron deficiencies can produce atrophic glossitis.

*Geographical tongue* is probably associated with one or other of the above conditions together with a local area of trauma from a tooth or denture. Fissuring of the tongue is an inherited characteristic.

*Varicosity* of the vessels on the under-surface of the tongue is due to age changes in the supportive connective tissues.

Other tongue changes may be due to mouth breathing and difficulty in swallowing or an unwillingness to swallow tablets which, unless nurses are vigilant, may lie in the mouth for long periods and cause irritation.

*Dental hygiene* is important in old people and often neglected. It is not usually worthwhile trying to persuade an elderly person to wear a denture if he has been without one for many years. However, many dentures worn by the elderly are 25 to 40 years old and are sometimes quite considerably damaged and often no longer fit properly either because of resorption of the gums with aging or occasionally because of cerebrovascular disease affecting the bulbar nuclei and thus the muscles of the tongue and of mastication. Dentures should, therefore, be checked from time to time by the dentist.

It is generally thought that the sensation of taste and smell become less acute with advancing age and while this is probably true, it is not something which has been carefully assessed.

*Acute parotitis* is a secondary condition often found in ill old people. It is due to ascending infection from the mouth. Sometimes it is associated with the terminal stage of an illness but if this is not the case, then its occurrence indicates the need for antibiotic treatment.

## Dysphagia

Dysphagia is a very important problem in old age and may be due to:

>    disorder of the nervous control of swallowing
>    pressure from outside the oesophagus
>    intrinsic disease of the oesophagus.

*Neurological causes.* As is the case with all other motile viscera of the body, neurological causes of oesophageal dysfunction are important in old age. They may be due to disease within the brain or autonomic nerves or age change in the neuromuscular system. The common neurological disorders in the elderly which lead to dysphagia are: stroke, bulbar palsy and presbyoesophagus.

In *stroke* the difficulty lies in transferring food from the mouth to the oesophagus. Sometimes fluid is regurgitated through the nose.

In *motor neurone disease* and *pseudo-bulbar palsy*, the difficulty may lie either in transferring the food bolus from the mouth to the oesophagus or there may be diffuse oesophageal spasm. While these two conditions produce similar effects, they are of quite different aetiology. Pseudobulbar palsy is associated with bilateral cerebrovascular disease of the brain stem and produces a small spastic tongue and exaggerated jaw jerk. Bulbar palsy due to motor neurone disease affects the bulbar nuclei themselves and produces fasciculation of the tongue. Both conditions may produce dysarthria and neurological signs of damage to the pyramidal tracts.

Age changes include *presbyoesophagus*, i.e. diffuse oesophageal spasm. Barium swallow shows a 'corkscrew oesophagus' or alternatively a simple loss of peristalsis. Presbyoesophagus has been reported particularly in 90-year-old people.

*Obstruction of the oesophagus from without.* Occasionally this may result from aneurysm of the aorta or marked tortuosity of the great vessels associated with arteriosclerosis; it may also be due to carcinoma particularly to metastatic deposits in mediastinal lymph glands. An oesophageal pouch, which fills with food, may produce dysphagia by pressure on the oesophagus. It is characterized by regurgitation of undigested food—sometimes hours after swallowed.

*Dysphagia arising from disease of the oesophagus itsef.* Here the possibilities are numerous but in old age first thought must be given to: (a) carcinoma (which unfortunately is usually well advanced before it causes oesophageal obstruction); (b) reflux oesophagitis, possibly leading to stricture and which may or may not be associated with hiatus hernia; (c) achalasia of the cardia; (d) moniliasis.

Other possible causes include stricture as a result of swallowing corrosive substances, scleroderma, impaction of a food bolus at the lower end of the oesophagus, and the Kelly-Paterson syndrome of epithelial webs at the upper end of the oesophagus in patients with iron deficiency anaemia.

Investigation should include not only a barium swallow but also oesophagoscopy with the flexible oesophagoscope. Oesophageal varices do not usually cause dysphagia, but they do occur in old people with hepatic cirrhosis.

Treatment of these conditions in the elderly is exactly the same as in younger people and since swallowing is such a basic function in life every effort must be made to overcome dysphagia in the elderly, unless it is clearly part of the very last stage of a terminal illness.

## Hiatus hernia

Hiatus hernia is a common concomitant of aging. It can cause a great deal of pain and discomfort but is often quite asymptomatic. It may cause prolonged occult bleeding over many months or many years leading eventually to an iron deficiency anaemia and is occasionally the site of a peptic ulcer. Since hiatus hernia is so common in old age (in one series it was reported as being present in 70 per cent of the over 70's) symptoms and complications cannot always be attributed to it simply because they co-exist. This problem is very similar to that of colonic diverticulosis and of cervical spondylosis, all common conditions in old age and in all of which symptoms may be attributed to them which are due to other causes.

Hiatus hernias may be either:

> *sliding;* this is the usual type in the elderly, associated with reflux oesophagitis and it is now generally thought that fibrosis following oesophagitis causes traction of the cardiac end of the stomach through the diaphragm
> *paraoesophageal* (or rolling hiatus hernia); this occurs no more often in the old than in the young. It is due to a herniation of part of the fundus of the stomach alongside the oesophagus through the diaphragm.

While there are other types of diaphragmatic hernia (e.g. Morgagni hernia—the movement of coils of the large bowel into the thorax through a defect in the attachment of the diaphragmatic fibres to the anterior chest wall), the sliding and paraoesophageal are the only two types of hiatus hernia. They may co-exist—a mixed hiatus hernia.

The sliding hiatus hernia produces substernal burning pain (due to oesophagitis) present especially when the patient stoops down or lies flat. Pain is often absent and the patient presents with anaemia due to occult bleeding. The condition is not easily treated by diet and the mainstay of the treatment is the frequent taking of antacids, if necessary, every hour. Magnesium trisilicate and aluminium hydroxide will not produce alkalosis and are the most satisfactory drugs to use. The patient should sleep with several pillows and possibly with the head of the bed raised on the blocks and should, as far as possible, avoid stooping down. If the pain is intractable then surgical treatment may have to be considered. This is a serious operation and must be approached with caution in the elderly.

*Age changes in gastric secretion*

There is an increasing frequency of gastric secretion failure and achlorhydria with advancing age.

## Peptic ulcer

The most striking difference in peptic ulceration between the old and the young is the frequent occurrence of asymptomatic benign giant gastric ulcer in old people; often an autopsy diagnosis. While this ulcer is often asymptomatic and therefore undiagnosed it is, nevertheless, a not unimportant cause of death. Altogether about one-third of all gastric ulcer deaths occur in the elderly.

The symptoms are likely to be general rather than specific and include anaemia, weight loss and vague upper abdominal pain. As in other conditions of the stomach and oesophagus, when an ulcer is suspected there should be no hesitation in requesting a gastroscopy with a flexible gastroscope, although it is usual to have barium studies carried out first.

The treatment of gastric ulcer has been revolutionized by the introduction of carbenoxolone sodium ('Biogastrone') and this should usually be given a trial before surgical operation is decided upon. In old people regular electrolyte surveillance and monitoring of blood pressure are important since carbenoxolone sodium often causes fluid retention, hypokalaemia and a rise in blood pressure. Thiazide diuretics and potassium supplementation may both be needed as ancillary therapeutic measures.

## Diverticulosis

As is apparent in other hollow organs, the development of

diverticula in the alimentary canal seems to be an age-related phenomenon. They are found in the oesophagus, duodenum and jejunum. In the duodenum some may be secondary to healed ulcers. In the small bowel they are often multiple. Multiple diverticula may be associated with vitamin $B_{12}$ deficiency.

## Pancreatitis

The occurrence of pancreatitis increases with age although it still remains a relatively rare condition. It is sometimes associated with accidental hypothermia. It is possible that ischaemia secondary to vascular disease has some part to play in this increased frequency of pancreatitis in the elderly.

### The malabsorption sydrome

The villi of the mucosa of the small bowel change their shape as they age, becoming shorter and broader. Since this means a diminution of absorbing surface it must be considered along with other factors which impair intestinal absorption.

*The xylose absorption test* is one of the standard methods of assessing intestinal absorption. In this test a standard dose of xylose is given orally and absorption is judged by the levels of urinary excretion of xylose over the next five hours. This test, therefore, depends not only on absorption from the small bowel but also on renal function, and it is unreliable in old age because renal function is quite often impaired to some degree. One method of circumventing this is to compare the urinary levels when xylose is given (a) by mouth and (b) intravenously. Another problem in the practical use of this test is that it is quite often difficult to obtain satisfactory samples of urine over a fixed period of time from old people either because of incontinence or difficulty with micturition or else because of a large residual urine which dilutes newly secreted urine containing the various chemical markers. The other standard test for the assessment of malabsorption is the three day collection of faeces and measurement for faecal fat. Collection of adequate faecal samples may present problems because of constipation and occasionally incontinence. The third method of diagnosis is by small bowel biopsy and with adequate premedication this can usually be carried out satisfactorily in even the very old.

One reason why the diagnosis of malabsorption is important in old people is because deficiency states (e.g. of folic acid, vitamin $B_{12}$, calcium and iron, and vitamin D) commonly result from malabsorption.

Other conditions in the upper alimentary tract do not vary greatly in their presentation and management in the old and the young and need not be dealt with here. They are, nonetheless, important and particularly carcinoma of the stomach which is one of the commonest forms of neoplasia in the over-85's. It should also be emphasized that perforation of a peptic ulcer with *acute peritonitis* may present a completely different clinical picture in old people and indeed is sometimes entirely asymptomatic and discovered only at autopsy: in particular the severe pain which is characteristic of this condition in younger people is often absent. Peritonitis must therefore be considered as a diagnostic possibility in all forms of acute generalized disease. Tenderness on palpation is not always present and more stress must therefore be laid on a previous history of dyspepsia, although even this is sometimes absent. The leucocyte count will be raised and usually pyrexia will be present. Sometimes the condition presents as an acute confusional state.

## The large bowel

### Bowel habit

Although old people as a group seem to be more aware of their bowel habit than younger people and more concerned about constipation, there is no evidence to suggest that in normal old people bowel habit is different from that in the young. Two surveys have been carried out among representative portions of the population including the elderly and these suggest that the normal range of bowel habit lies between three motions a day and three a week and that this is the same at all age groups. Nevertheless, old people take laxatives more often than do the young and this may seem to indicate a propensity to constipation. However, it may only indicate the fact that most people who are now old were brought up at the beginning of this century to believe that regular purgation was essential to health because of the theories of auto-intoxication from the constipated colon.

## Constipation

Though bowel habit is the same in the old as in the young, constipation is an important accompaniment of debility and, therefore, the problem of constipation in old age requires special consideration.

Constipation may mean one of two things, either *difficult defaecation*, possibly because of hardness of stool but occurring with the normal regularity, or else a change in bowel habit so that *defaecation becomes less frequent*. It is important to discover which of these two conditions the patient may be complaining of since each may indicate a different cause. Indeed, it is possible for an old person to have a bowel motion every day and still to be constipated.

The consistency of the stool is likely to be related to diet and to intestinal transit time, i.e. time taken for material which is swallowed to appear in the stool. In general, a high residue diet will be associated with a normal intestinal transit time and easily passed, well-formed stools. Transit time is dependent not only on diet but also on the mobility of the patient. It is in the immobile old person that transit time may be very much prolonged and as a result of this stools may become hard and difficult to pass.

Transit times through the gut are measured by giving the patient appropriate markers to take by mouth and by noting the period of time that is required for 80 per cent of the markers to be passed rectally. The most convenient way of doing this is to use small capsules filled with barium and to monitor their presence by radiographs. In a normal person of any age, 80 per cent of the markers will be cleared within 72 hours. In disabled (and therefore immobile) old people, the period of time taken for 80 per cent of the markers to be passed can be in excess of seven days. Constipation is, therefore, a particular menace in immobile old people and is one of the important reasons why every attempt must be made to maintain some form of exercise and mobility among the elderly disabled.

Constipation has a number of other important causes in old

age, notable among which are depression, carcinoma of the large bowel, hypoparathyroidism and the effect of some drugs such as iron. If constipation presents as a recent change in bowel habit then the possibility of a malignant growth in the colon or rectum is important.

The treatment of constipation requires in the first place the diagnosis and treatment of its underlying cause, with special reference to diet and mobility. However, it is not always possible to enable a disabled old person to take regular exercise and in such a person high residue diet alone may not help the situation. Therefore, regular treatment in such cases with either purgatives, suppositories or enemas is good medical practice.

*The classification of the purgatives (see Table 14.1)*

Table 14.1  Classification of the purgatives

---

*Bulk*
    Bran
    Agar
    Mucilaginous gums
    Salines

*Lubricant*
    Liquid paraffin
    Dioctyl sodium sulphosuccinate   }
    Poloxalkol              }     'Stool softeners'

*Irritant*
Anthracenes: Senna
              Cascara
    Bisacodyl
    Phenolphthalein

*Other*
    Normacol—changing flora of lower bowel by alteration of pH

---

*Bulk purgatives.* As indicated above, bran is a 'natural' bulk purgative and can be used to increase the residue of the diet either by taking bread made from unrefined flour (wheatmeal bread), or by sprinkling powdered bran on the food. Other bulk purgatives include Agar and a number of hydrophilic gums, but these are not recommended for use in immobile old people.

Saline purgatives cause the retention of large quantities of fluid in the bowel by their hydrophilic qualities. This large bulk leads to stimulation of peristalsis and bowel emptying. They may thus be called bulk purgatives, although their action is short lived. They should only be used in the elderly to produce an isolated bowel emptying (as in preparation for an X-ray) and not regularly used.

Lubricant purgatives include liquid paraffin and a number of the so-called 'stool softeners'. Liquid paraffin is a popular purgative in this country but is not recommended in the elderly for the following reasons: it can cause inhalation lipid pneumonia because of difficulty in swallowing which occurs in some elderly people; it can absorb fat soluble vitamins and, therefore, predispose to osteomalacia; it can leak from the anus. The so-called 'faecal softeners' lower the surface tension of faeces and thus allow the penetration of water. They include dioctyl sodium sulphosuccinate and poloxalkol and are ingredients in a number of widely used combination purgatives.

The third and most widely used group of purgatives in the elderly are the irritant purgatives. In the past this group has included a whole range of pharmacological agents which were sold under the guise of 'vegetable purgatives'. Nowadays there are two main groups in use: the anthracenes and the drug bisacodyl. Their pharmacological action is slightly different. The anthracenes include cascara sagrada, senna and castor oil. These are absorbed from the small bowel, broken down in the liver to the active principle (emodin) which is excreted into the large bowel where it has an irritant effect on the myenteric plexuses. The most important member of this group nowadays is senna, available as a standardized preparation ('Senokot'). Bisacodyl on the other hand is not absorbed from the gut but has a direct stimulant effect on the myenteric plexuses and it may, therefore, be given either orally or rectally. Bisacodyl (marketed as 'Dulcolax') is available either in the form of tablets or of suppositories.

The combination of an anthracene purgative with a stool softener is popular in geriatric practice. Two examples are dioctyl sodium sulphosuccinate plus an anthracene purgative ('Normax') and poloxalkol plus an anthracene purgative ('Dorbanex'). The latter occasionally stains the perianal skin red.

*Suppositories.* Bisacodyl and glycerine suppositories are both popular with the elderly. Another type of suppository is one which releases carbon dioxide within the rectum and causes evacuation following rectal distension ('Beogex)'. Thus these three types of suppository all have different actions.

*Enemas.* Large bulk soap and water enemas are no longer recommended in old people, partly because of the possibility of producing shock as a result of rapid rectal distension, and partly because of the possibility of rupturing a colonic diverticulum. Small bulk phosphate enemas, however, are very suitable. They contain 130 ml of hygroscopic substances such as sodium acid phosphate and sodium phosphate. These phosphate enemas are conveniently presented in disposable packages but care must always be taken not to traumatize the anal canal.

*Choice of treatment.* The type of treatment depends on the type of constipation. The most severe form of constipation is associated with faecal impaction in which the long standing presence of faeces in the sigmoid colon and rectum has led to the development of hard, impacted masses which will, if large enough, require digital breakdown before being passed. However, this is an unpleasant procedure both for the patient and for the person who carries it out (a doctor rather than a nurse) and if possible attempts to soften the mass and have it evacuated by the use of a stool softener together with enemas or suppositories should be tried first. In this situation irritant purgatives are not recommended since they are likely to cause faecal incontinence. In severe constipation, therefore, the objective must be to have the whole rectum and colon emptied by suppositories or by enemas, a procedure which is likely to require the use of these agents every day for seven to ten days. It must be emphasized that securing one evacuation from the lower bowel of a constipated old person is not sufficient, as only the rectum is likely to be emptied and further masses of firm or hard faeces will quickly move round from the rest of the colon. Diligent daily treatment is required therefore until the enema is returned without any result and clinical examination indicates that the rectum and colon are empty.

Once constipation has been completely dealt with in this way, it must be considered whether prevention of its recurrence is necessary. If constipation has resulted from the patient's immobility and if the immobility remains, then some additional treatment is needed to prevent recurrence of the constipation. This may be either the use of a combined stool softener and anthracene purgative or of standardized senna or of regular suppositories or enemas given once or twice a week. It may indeed be a combination of two of these methods. The most appropriate treatment, its frequency and dosage, will vary from individual to individual.

The advantage of a small enema or of suppositories is that a result is obtained within a short period of time and the attendant can be sure of their effectiveness. A disadvantage is that they usually require to be given by a nurse. The irritant purgatives on the other hand have the disadvantage that they can cause faecal incontinence in old people. A number of long-term effects of the use of regular anthracene purgatives have been described (e.g. degeneration of Auerbach's plexus) but it seems unlikely that these are important among the elderly. As least this has not yet been demonstrated.

## Megacolon

Idiopathic megacolon occurs more commonly among old people than among the young and also more commonly among immobile and institutionalized populations than among those at home. There are probably several factors involved in its production (e.g. immobility leading to long-standing constipation, the use of anticholinergic drugs (e.g. in Parkinsonism) and possibly, although this has still to be shown, age changes affecting the peripheral autonomic plexuses). Idiopathic megacolon often presents with faecal incontinence and may be suspected from the considerable distension of the abdomen with gas. It is not an easy condition to treat. The first approach is usually the treatment of constipation and the second approach is the use of either neostigmine or other cholinergic drugs such as mebervine. Occasionally it leads to intestinal obstruction due to volvulus of the sigmoid colon. Sometimes the volvulus will be corrected following sigmoidoscopy, but over 50 per cent of cases require operative surgical treatment.

**Other diseases of the colon which are important in the elderly**

*Diverticular disease*

The development of colonic diverticula becomes more common with increasing age. They are almost never found in the young but in Western society are found in about 20 per cent of normal people between the ages of 50 and 60, 30 per cent of those between 60 and 80 and 40 per cent of people aged over 80. This development of colonic diverticula with age is not found in other cultures throughout the world and is thought to be associated with the low residue diet which has become a feature of life in Western society. There is a striking geographical difference between diverticular disease in Western countries and its rarity in countries such as Africa and the Far East. Further evidence which relates it to a low residue diet is the fact that during the 1939–45 War, when the national loaf containing a portion of unrefined flour was in use in Great Britain, the incidence of diverticulitis dropped and that, by contrast, this disease was only reported with any frequency from the beginning of the twentieth century when widespread use of refined flour became common. Finally, it has been shown that rats fed on a low residue diet develop colonic diverticula whereas those on a normal residue diet do not.

Since colonic diverticula commonly develop as an accompaniment of aging, great caution must be observed in attributing to diverticular disease the development of bowel symptoms. The demonstration of colonic diverticula on a barium enema is not in itself sufficient evidence in old people that their symptoms are due to this cause.

The reason why low residue diet should predispose to the development of diverticula has been explained by Painter as follows:

At the recto-sigmoid junction there is a functional sphincter which results from the contraction of the transverse muscles of the colon forming the normal colonic haustrations. The areas between haustrations have been compared to bladders by Painter and the greater the quantity of transverse muscle contraction, the higher the pressure within the bladders. Since this area acts as a functional sphincter, then the less bulky are the colonic contents, so the greater frequency of contractions will be required to prevent the onward passage of this faeces to the rectum. On the other hand, the more bulky the faeces, the less contraction needed. Thus in patients on a high residue diet there is likely to be evolved less high pressure within the 'bladders' of the colon (see Fig. 14.1)—and so less likelihood of diverticula developing.

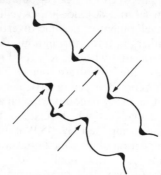

Fig. 14.1 'Bladdering' in the sigmoid colon resulting in colonic diverticulum.

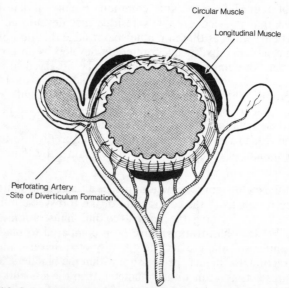

Fig. 14.2 Cross-section of the colon indicating diverticulum formation.

Another important factor, is the strength of the colon wall itself. Diverticula develop between the colonic taenia, particularly at the weak spot where the perforating arteries pass through the colonic wall (Fig. 14.2). It is likely that the strength of the colonic wall is impaired with advancing age because of diminished elasticity within connective tissues, and this together with the increased pressure within the segments of the colon lead to the development of diverticula.

*Symptoms.* Colonic diverticula may be present without producing any symptoms at all and they are only seen if looked for by barium enema. Pain occurs in about 78 per cent of patients who have been diagnosed as suffering from diverticular disease. Pain may be present for two reasons; in the first place as a result of a colic due to muscle spasm as described above and secondly, as a result of inflammation. The pain itself is not diagnostic of diverticulitis and it may often be relieved by antispasmodic treatment such as the anticholinergic drug, propantheline.

Pain and tenderness in the left iliac fossa are characteristic of diverticular disease. Change in bowel habit is another important symptom but this may be either with the development of diarrhoea or of constipation and of these two, constipation is the more common. Some patients develop alternating constipation and diarrhoea. The third important symptom is rectal bleeding which occurs in about 30 per cent of patients in whom a diagnosis of diverticular disease has been made. Urinary symptoms, due to an inflammatory area contiguous to the bladder, occurs in a smaller number. Other alimentary tract symptoms such as nausea, flatulence and vomiting are also common. On examination there is sometimes a palpable mass in the left iliac fossa and usually this is tender. Alternatively a tender mass may be palpated rectally.

The important complications of diverticular disease are those of infection (diverticulitis and abscess formation possibly going on to the formation of fistulae) and perforation which may lead to peritonitis. Occasionally there may be intestinal obstruction.

In all but the most acute cases, treatment involves a high residue diet and the use of antispasmodic drugs such as propantheline. In acute cases a fluid diet must be instituted and the drug pethidine may be required to control symptoms. Morphine should never be used in this disease since it will increase the motility of the colon and aggravate the underlying causative mechanism. Diverticulitis must be treated by anti-biotics and if these are not successful then by surgery. Occasionally the formation of a colostomy is necessary to control symptoms.

## Carcinoma of the colon and rectum

Cancer of the alimentary tract is one of the commonest causes of death in old age and with any change in bowel habit, carcinoma of the colon and rectum must be considered. If carcinoma is suspected and cannot be diagnosed by rectal examination, a sigmoidoscopy must be carried out and followed by a barium enema. It is sometimes argued that these measures are expensive and disagreeable and should not be used in old age to make the diagnosis of malignant disease if surgery is not going to be used. While there are occasions when this argument is appropriate, in general it is essential to establish a diagnosis at any age since treatable conditions may always be found and in any case the management of terminal malignant disease can be embarked on with much more confidence if the diagnosis is certain. The surgical cure rate for carcinoma of the colon without lymph node involvement is 80 per cent (with 5 years survival).

## Ischaemic colitis

Since one of the features of old age is the development of atherosclerotic vascular disease, it might be anticipated that ischaemic colitis would be a condition as common as transient cerebral ischaemia and ischaemic heart disease. However, this is not the case and the reason for this is probably the nature of the blood supply to the large bowel. This is shown in Fig. 14.3, where it may be clearly seen that the two major blood vessels, the superior mesenteric and inferior mesenteric arteries divide first into a number of major branches and that these in turn supply the gut through a series of arcades—being all linked together by a marginal artery. The marginal artery thus provides a major anastomotic channel and for this reason minor degrees of ischaemia in the colon are relatively uncom-

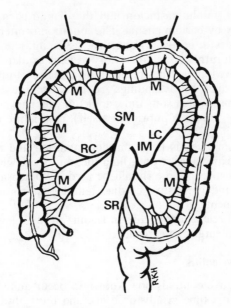

Fig. 14.3 Blood supply to the colon. SM, superior mesenteric; IM, inferior mesenteric; RC, right colic; LC, left colic; SR, superior rectal; M, marginal.

mon, although major gangrene due to obstruction of the superior or inferior mesenteric arteries themselves is an occasional surgical emergency in the elderly. Ischaemic colitis, however, does occur and must always be suspected in a patient presenting with episodes of abdominal pain, diarrhoea and blood in the stool. The most vulnerable area of the colon is the splenic flexure for there is the extremity of the blood supply of the two major arteries.

Very often there is a precipitating cause to the attack of ischaemic colitis—such as a drop in blood pressure or an episode of dehydration. Congestive cardiac failure may also precipitate it and the use of digitalis may be implicated although it is not entirely clear whether this is a precipitating cause separate from the congestive cardiac failure for which the drug is being used. The condition usually occurs suddenly and may be associated with an intense fear of food. Abdominal pain and loose stools containing red blood or blood clot confirm the suspicion and the diagnosis can be made definitely by barium enema. The condition is often transitory since, as with cerebral ischaemia, tissue infarction does not occur but rather an inflammatory oedema exudate which may be followed after it has resolved by a degree of fibrous tissue scarring. The X- ray findings are, therefore, those of an area of oedema (which sometimes looks on the barium enema as though a thumb is imprinting itself). A stricture may be the end result.

Ischaemic colitis is a transient condition and therefore is treated expectantly with a fluid diet and if analgesics are required then pethidine should be used. Hypotension must be treated and congestive cardiac failure requires appropriate management.

Mesenteric artery occlusion leading to infarction and gangrene is a surgical emergency.

### Ulcerative colitis

Ulcerative colitis is now known to occur quite commonly for the first time in advanced age and must always be considered in the diagnosis of disorders of the lower bowel in the elderly. The condition presents with a change in bowel habit, particularly with diarrhoea, the stool often being blood-stained and mucus containing. Severe diarrhoea may lead to dehydration and collapse: bleeding may lead to anaemia. The diagnosis and management of this condition is the same in old age as it is in younger people.

A less severe, simple granular proctitis occasionally presents as diarrhoea or faecal incontinence in old age. It is not associated with blood in the stool and sigmoidoscopy shows a uniform hyperaemic velvety appearance of the rectal mucosa. This condition is usually treated very successfully by a series of retention enemas of hydrocortisone hemisuccinate given once or twice a day. Retention of the enema is sometimes aided by giving a dose of propantheline half an hour before the enema and also by elevating the foot of the bed.

### Differential diagnosis of disease of the lower bowel in old age

Pain, diarrhoea and faecal incontinence require a careful

differential diagnosis including the conditions mentioned above as well as Crohn's disease (which tends particularly and in distinction to the others to affect the anus and peri-anal region and which may have the typical appearance on barium examination of discreet areas of involvement of the bowel—the so-called 'string sign').

# 15. Electrolyte and Body Fluid Disorders

The idea that the body fluids provide a kind of internal sea of serene composition in which cells may safely bathe, was generated in the mid-nineteenth century by the French physiologist Claude Bernard. Later, an American physiologist, Walter Cannon coined the word 'homeostasis' and developed the notion that the body has homeostatic mechanisms specially designed to preserve the steady state, whatever the environment outside the body.

Water comprises about 56 per cent of the body weight; there are about 80 pints in an 11 stone man. This water is in two 'compartments'; one third comprises the *extracellular* fluid (ECF) and two thirds is inside cells, the *intracellular* fluid (ICF). The ICF is, in fact, the sum total of all the minute amounts of water inside the millions of body cells, but its composition is uniform enough for it to be regarded, for thinking purposes, as a large freely communicating pool.

The electrolyte make-up of the cell's fluid is different from that of ECF; potassium ion ($K^+$) predominates inside cells while sodium ($Na^+$) is the chief ion of the ECF. This difference in composition is kept up by the cell membrane which is not merely an inert, porous bag, but exerts a complicated biochemical 'pumping' action involving an expulsion of $Na^+$ from the cell and $K^+$ transport into it.

Two important ideas to grasp are:

1. Both the chemical make-up *and* the volume of the ECF and ICF are kept steady. The means for achieving these two ends are however, only partly separate: for example the kidney can alter the excretion of water or of electrolytes depending on which is threatened, but compromises between keeping salt or volume constant are often necessary.

2. Though the patterns of chemical make-up of ICF and

ECF differ very much, the *total solute concentration* of the two fluids is always equal. If, for any reason, solute is selectively lost from or introduced into only one of the two fluid compartments, water will move in whatever direction tends to restore osmotic equality.

## The changes in homeostasis with advancing age

Advancing age does not bring in its wake any intrinsic changes in the steady state conditions, but it does bring a reduced capacity of the homeostatic responses necessary when the internal sea is threatened by metabolic storms.

The most important of the organs involved, the kidney, loses functional ability steadily throughout life; by the age of 90 years both the creatinine and the PAH clearances have fallen to about half the level at age 30. The essential consequence is a fall in the maximum possible solute concentration of urine. Another organ involved in homeostatic responses, the lung, also shows progressive loss of function as age advances, and its compensatory powers also become limited.

## Clinical disturbances

A catalogue of the host of conditions which can influence water and electrolyte metabolism would make soporific reading, so the following account deals selectively with a small number of familiar situations in geriatric practice:

1. Water depletion
2. 'Low sodium syndromes', including electrolyte depletion in intestinal disease and after surgical operation
3. Potassium depletion.

## Water depletion

This term is used in preference to 'dehydration' which is often loosely used to mean either a pure water loss or loss of salt and water together; these two disorders require different treatment and should be kept separate in the mind.

In health the total body water is kept constant over any appreciable period of time by adjusting the amount of liquid drunk to equal the losses in urine, breath and sweat. The fluid input is controlled by *thirst*, a sensation known to all.

The slaking of thirst is an activity taken for granted by

healthy, alert adults; we feel thirst, we know what the sensation means and we take steps to remove it by getting fluid ourselves (or getting others to do if for us) and then we drink. The relief of thirst due to water depletion is pleasurable, while there are more hedonistic reasons for drinking than the quenching of thirst for purely biological reasons.

Though normal people slake thirst more or less unthinkingly, the water balance of ill, old people is often jeopardised because they fail in one or more of the four steps mentioned above:

1.  Thirst sensation can be blunted
2.  Although the patient is aware of the thirst sensation, there is recognition neither of its meaning nor of the action required
3.  Even when perception of thirst sensation, its significance and the action required are normal, fluid may not be accessible because action is impeded by immobility due to apathy, stupor, or physical limitation of movement
4.  When all else, perception of thirst and the correct 'biological response' are normal, mechanical difficulties of swallowing may reduce fluid intake.

The patients most at risk of water depletion are the mentally confused, those in coma or stupor and those with febrile general illness. Water depletion itself can cause mental disturbances and will 'compound confusion' if any already exists.

*Water depletion often goes unrecognized.* The sufferers may be unable to express their needs, and the signs of water lack are inconspicuous, but, like all diagnoses, water depletion is easy to recognize, and to correct, once the possibility is considered. It is important to keep water lack in mind in any old person who has been:

Comatose or stuporose for more than 24 hours
Immobilized in isolation for any reason
Demented or confused with breakdown of social organization.

The physical signs of water depletion are unimpressive until the condition is severe. The skin is dry, but has not the same lack of turgor (juiciness) that characterizes loss of both salt and water. Likewise, the tongue is dry, and furred because the patient is lethargic and does not eat. The blood pressure does not fall, nor is there venous collapse as in salt depletion.

Confirmation of the diagnosis of water depletion is simply obtained: a venous blood sample will show increased concentrations of the serum electrolyte values, e.g. the serum sodium can be raised to 155 to 160 mEq per 1 (normal 139 $\pm$ 2 and the potassium level to 5 to 6 mEq per l. The rate of urine flow is low but the urine is highly coloured and its specific gravity high. The blood urea is often raised and can be very high in severe water lack.

## Treatment

The treatment is simple: (1) free access to water and encouragement to drink in those who are mentally clear and not physically prevented from drinking; (2) free, easy access to water and *supervision that adequate drinking actually occurs* in the confused (it is useless to leave a water jug by the bedside) and (3) infusions of isotonic dextrose intravenously in those who are stuporose, comatose or physically prevented from drinking. The dextrose (50 g per l) will usually provide enough calories to prevent any gross catabolic changes occurring while the water depletion is being repaired.

The total amount of fluid needed for replacement can be roughly gauged from the formula:

$$\text{Vol } (\ell) = \frac{(\text{serum Na (mEq per } \ell ) - 140) \times \text{body weight (kg)}}{200}$$

e.g. 50 kg patient with a serum sodium of 156 mEq/$\ell$ would require 4 litres of fluid.

Once the water deficit has been made up, a conscious patient will regulate automatically his own fluid intake.

## 'Low sodium syndromes'

A common problem in geriatric patients is the finding of a low serum sodium concentration: the normal value is 139 $\pm$ 2 mEq per l and values of 132 mEq per l or less qualify as 'hyponatraemia'.

Table 15.1 below lists the common causes of hyponatraemia; the first two of which are the most important.

Table 15.1 Common causes of hyponatraemia

1. True sodium depletion
2. The quartet of a low serum sodium concentration, oedema resistant to diuretics, persistent congestive heart failure and pre-renal uraemia
3. Iatrogenic water excess      ⎫ causing
4. Excessive ADH effect from certain  ⎬ 'dilutional'
    neoplasms                ⎭ hyponatraemia
5. Hyponatraemia of unknown mechanism occurring in the course of severe general disease

## 1. *True sodium depletion*

By 'true sodium depletion' is meant a state in which the total sodium content of the body has fallen. Loss of sodium inevitably entails some water loss, the brunt of which falls on the ECF and plasma with relatively little change in ICF volume. The clinical signs are dominated by four factors: reduced turgor of the subcutaneous tissues due to depletion of interstitial fluid; the circulatory effects of reduction in plasma volume; the intrinsic 'water intoxication' effects of a low serum sodium concentration, and any attendant acid-base disturbances.

Loss of tissue turgor gives rise to a gaunt, desiccated, general appearance; the eyes are sunken and eyeball tension is low. Dryness and furring of the tongue and lips make speech and chewing difficult. The skin is lank, and when a fold on the limbs or abdomen is pinched up between the examiner's fingers, it remains deformed for longer than normal.

Circulatory examination reveals collapsed jugular veins and the signs of reduced cardiac output: the peripheral pulse is of small volume and the blood pressure is subnormal, often with a large orthostatic fall. In more advanced sodium lack, with gross reduction of blood volume, there is intense peripheral vasoconstriction with cold, cyanotic extremities and a very low blood pressure.

Although in the early stages of sodium depletion water loss almost keeps pace with electrolyte loss in an attempt to preserve normal serum osmolarity, water loss lags behind when sodium depletion continues unabated for long; then the serum sodium concentration falls more steeply and the signs of 'water intoxication' set in. Mental confusion, to which the enfeebled old are always vulnerable, often appears first. Muscle cramps and myoclonic or epileptiform seizures occur, but are rarely prominent in old people; these signs are seen at their most intense in the sodium depletion associated with heat exhaustion in younger adults.

Sodium depletion is often only one element in a severe metabolic disturbance, especially when it is provoked by an intestinal catastrophe. Acid-base disturbances are often present and depletion of $K^+$ can also co-exist with sodium lack, so measurement of the blood pH and $pCO_2$ and estimates of the serum potassium and bicarbonate ion levels are necessary if one is to understand and treat the metabolic disturbance comprehensively.

*Causes.* The causes of sodium depletion in old people are much the same as in younger adults. The common ones are:

*Loss of upper intestinal secretions*
Small bowel obstruction with vomiting
Therapeutic aspiration of small bowel contents
Fistulae between the small and large bowels (including jejunostomy and ileostomy)
*Severe watery diarrhoea*
Acute gastroenteritis
Specific, acute, bacterial infections of the large bowel (bacillary dysentery, cholera, etc.)
Iatrogenic: staphylococcal enteritis caused by some broad spectrum antibiotics, especially tetracycline, chlortetracycline and clindamycin
Excessive purgation by laxatives or magnesium sulphate
Forced diuresis from potent diuretics or ion exchange resins (see below)
severe therapeutic dietary sodium restriction: the 'rice diet'
*Renal loss of sodium*
Chronic 'salt-losing' nephritis
Sudden relief of urinary obstruction
Osmotic diuresis: diabetic coma, recovery from acute nephritis, etc.

## 2. *Congestive heart failure*

This is very common in old people and a 'low sodium syndrome' is a frequent, knotty therapeutic problem which crops up after prolonged treatment with potent diuretics.

In this state, although the serum sodium concentration is often greatly lowered, the circulatory response to the diuretics dwindles steadily until there is at last persistent jugular venous congestion, often with functional tricuspid valve incompetence, coupled with intractable peripheral oedema and venous engorgement of the liver.

The mechanisms responsible for this state have never been fully explained, but the effects on renal haemodynamics are probably the main basis for it. The cardiac output is low and this diminishes glomerular filtration and renal perfusion, as a result of which the blood urea rises, often exceeding 100 mg per 100 ml.

Emergence of this clinical picture usually has a sinister prognostic meaning. Ringing the changes between the potent diuretics which inhibit sodium re-absorption in the proximal limb of the distal renal tubule (frusemide, the thiazides and ethacrynic acid) rarely gives much benefit, and a switch to diuretics such as spironolactone which inhibit aldosterone's sodium-conserving action usually gives only a temporary improvement.

## 3. *Iatrogenic water excess*

In this condition there is no loss of sodium from the body, but excess water is introduced, usually in the course of misconceived or ill-controlled parenteral therapy. Water intoxication is only likely to occur when non-saline fluids are being given by either intravenous or rectal infusion to patients who are in stupor or coma and therefore unable to protest. In postoperative situations an additional factor is the reduction of urine flow caused by ADH secreted in response to pain or morphine.

The first symptoms are mental confusion, malaise, headache and nausea; the signs are puffiness of the face and oedema of the ankles. If overhydration is persisted with convulsions and death can result.

The condition can be avoided by frequent measurements of

the serum sodium concentration and haematocrit in all patients receiving infusions other than normal saline, e.g. '4 per cent dextrose with 1/5 normal saline'. When signs of water intoxication have actually appeared, the infusion must be stopped, then if urine flow is rapid and the hyponatraemia is mild, the condition will probably correct itself. Otherwise hypertonic saline (5 per cent sodium chloride) should be given, either by repeated injections of 100 ml or by intravenous infusion; to avoid tacking from one extreme of serum sodium concentration to the other, frequent control blood measurements are needed.

4. *Excessive ADH effect from neoplasms*

Occasionally, a bronchial neoplasm (which can be quite inconspicuous of itself) secretes a polypeptide hormone with a water retaining, ADH-like effect. The condition is usually discovered by finding a low serum $[Na^+]$ on routine examination.

5. *Hyponatraemia*

In a proportion of patients with hyponatraemia no clearly defined cause will be found. Some presumably have what Black (1967) describes as 'new steady states', i.e. they respond normally to changes of salt intake and their condition is not improved by hypertonic saline. Others, at the end of their lives, can have a generalized breakdown of the mechanism in cell membranes which maintains the electrolyte pattern of ICF against a gradient—the 'sick cell syndrome'. Yet others possibly entail a disturbance of the 'set-point' of osmotic receptors in the hypothalamus.

## Potassium depletion

Deficiency of potassium is a common and important disorder in old people: common because many roads lead to deficiency of $K^+$, and important because the effects are serious and sometimes lethal, but often correctable.

*Physiology*

Potassium is the main 'anion' of intracellular fluid where it is present in a concentration of about 100 mEq per l. Its presence influences many enzyme reactions, so depletion of potassium below the optimal level causes severe functional disturbances; if the deficiency is prolonged and profound, irreversible organic changes eventually appear.

About 70 per cent of the body's potassium is inside skeletal muscle cells, so it is not surprising that the main brunt of $K^+$ deficiency falls on muscle; cardiac and intestinal smooth muscle are also affected.

Potassium is also present in the extracellular fluid (including plasma) and although the external concentration is much lower—only 1/25th of the intracellular fluid level—it also has an important influence on impulse conduction and muscle contractibility. The 'resting membrane potential' of muscle cells is a function of the ratio between their intracellular and extracellular $K^+$ concentrations; irritability, i.e. the ease with which a contraction can be fired off, depends in turn on the membrane potential.

Potassium can move freely across the cell membrane, and redistribution of $K^+$ between the internal medium of cells and the extracellular fluid, without any depletion of total body $K^+$, can cause sudden functional disturbances. Acidosis causes $K^+$ to move out of cells into the ECF while alkalosis does the reverse. The most potent cause of an abrupt efflux of potassium out of the ECF, so reducing the serum $K^+$ concentration, is rapid absorption of a glucose load given together with insulin.

### Causes of potassium deficiency

The common causes of potassium depletion are listed as single items in Table 15.2 but it is important to remember that several different causes may be operating simultaneously to produce potassium depletion, also that a deficiency of $K^+$ is often merely one aspect of a complicated metabolic defect.

### Inadequate dietary intake

Young adults take from 50 to 150 mEq of potassium daily in their diet. Most old people have a potassium intake which is right at the lower end of this range and many teeter perpetually on the brink of potassium lack, since some degree of depletion is probably inevitable if the daily intake of $K^+$ falls below 25 to 35 mEq per day. A purely dietary deficiency develops slowly and is rarely the cause of severe symptoms,

Table 15.2 Some common causes of potassium depletion

---

*Inadequate dietary intake*
  Poor diet, isolation, poverty, apathy
*Diuretic therapy*
*Steroid therapy*
*Diarrhoea*
  Abuse of purgatives
  Ulcerative colitis
  Severe diverticulitis
  Steatorrhoea
  Villous papilloma of the colon
*Severe tissue injury or anoxia*
  Trauma
  Fracture
  Surgical operation
*Loss of intestinal secretions*
  Aspiration of intestinal contents
  Fistulae
  Vomiting

---

usually nothing more than mild impairment of muscular strength and general lethargy result. But this low-key potassium deficiency can set the scene for an unexpectedly severe effect when $K^+$ loss results from some acute disturbance such as diarrhoea or accidental trauma.

The typical daily 'external balance' of potassium of a healthy old person might be:

| Intake (mEq) | Output (mEq) |
|---|---|
| 55 | Stools 5 to 10 |
|  | Urine 45 to 50 |

The daily loss of 5 to 10 mEq in the stools does not represent nonabsorbed dietary potassium: it comes from $K^+$ secreted into the lumen of the large bowel. This loss is inevitable and continues even when there is $K^+$ depletion.

*Diuretics*

Congestive heart failure is so frequent in the elderly and the use of potent diuretics for its treatment so common that these drugs are now the chief offenders in causing potassium deficiency. All drugs of the thiazide class cause some degree of increased $K^+$ excretion in the urine as part of the price paid for a forced $Na^+$ excretion, and none can safely be given to old people without a separate oral supplement of potassium. An effective diuresis will often result in a negative balance of 20 to 30 mEq of $K^+$ per day. To offset this a *minimum* supplement of 1·8 g KCl (=about 24 mEq $K^+$) is needed daily (see p. 175).

### Diarrhoea

Potassium depletion can result not only from profuse watery diarrhoea as, for example, in acute gastroenteritis, but also from the passage of frequent, bulky but formed stools as in severe steatorrhoea.

Many old people believe that life cannot be good without at least one motion each day, and habitually flay their bowel into activity with the help of anthracene or phenolphthalein laxatives. These drugs are potent causes of potassium loss in the stool and can cause very severe though quietly developing potassium depletion. Ulcerative colitis in relapse can also cause fulminant $K^+$ deficiency.

### Loss of intestinal secretions

There is a large 'internal circuit' of potassium in the small intestine and pancreas, which daily secrete several litres of juice with a high potassium content. All the potassium so secreted is normally re-absorbed in the bowel and there is no net loss of potassium ion. However, the daily 'turnover' of $K^+$ in the intestinal lumen is about three times the total body content of potassium, so aspiration of even a small part of these intestinal secretions, or their loss from external or internal fistulae, can rapidly cause a massive loss of potassium.

Vomiting of gastric contents alone rarely causes severe potassium loss: the primary deficit is a loss of $H^+$ and $Cl^-$ which results in a metabolic alkalosis. This change in hydrion concentration causes K to move out of the ECF into cells and the serum K level falls as a result.

### Tissue trauma or anoxia

Oxygen lack or trauma to tissues, especially to skeletal muscle, causes potassium to move out of the cells into ECF. In the early stages this will merely cause a slightly elevated serum $K^+$ concentration, but because the quantity of potassium filtered at the glomerulus increases, so excretion in the urine rises and a depletion of the electrolyte eventually develops. Surgical operations, especially when performed on an old person who is already teetering for dietary reasons on the edge of $K^+$ deficiency are a frequent cause of sudden potassium depletion.

*Symptoms and signs of potassium depletion*

Experimentally induced depletion of potassium has shewn that depletion up to about 10 per cent of the body total, i.e. a loss of about 250 mEq in an old person, will cause no symptoms. At this level, and with more severe depletion, a material fall of plasma $K^+$ occurs only if the sodium intake is simultaneously high. It is of practical importance to realize that under some circumstances quite severe potassium depletion can exist without the serum $K^+$ concentration being unequivocally low.

The symptoms and signs of potassium deficiency, all, some or none of which can be present at any given serum $K^+$ level are:

1. Muscle weakness: this is often detectable in ill patients simply as severe general lethargy or mild weakness of the hand grip. In more severe states of $K^+$ depletion particular muscle groups can show complete paralysis

2. Mental confusion

3. Shallow, quick, irregular, 'fish-mouth' respiration

4. Abdominal distension: some degree of this is very common in $K^+$ deficiency, but in old people it is not so rarely the predominant sign. The presence of grossly dilated loops of large bowel can suggest idiopathic megacolon or raise suspicion of large bowel obstruction

5. Tetany occurs but is rare, except when hypokalaemia coexists with severe alkalosis (see below)

6. Cardiac arrhythmias and ECG changes. Electrocardiographic signs of $K^+$ deficiency are important for confirmation of clinical suspicion of potassium depletion, and as a warning that arrhythmia may occur. The ECG signs, in order of their evolution are: flattening of precordial T-waves with prolongation of the Q–T interval, the appearance of large U-waves, 'sagging' of the S–T segment producing a 'cove-plane' shape like that of digitalis intoxication, and finally fusion of the T- and U-waves. These changes are reasonably well correlated

with the serum $K^+$ value, and they are an indication of liability to the appearance of an arrhythmia—always a serious event in an old person.

The arrhythmia is usually paroxysmal atrial tachycardia with variable atrioventricular block ('PATB'): the chief danger lies in embarrassment of aged myocardial tissue by a fast ventricular rate.

### The biochemical findings in potassium depletion

The normal range for serum $K^+$ concentration is 3·5 to 5·0 mEq per litre; values in the range 2·0 to 3·5 are commonly seen in severe $K^+$ depletion, though it has already been emphasized that a normal serum $K^+$ does not by any means exclude significant and perhaps serious $K^+$ depletion.

In many instances of 'pure' K depletion, lowering of the serum $K^+$ concentration will be the only biochemical abnormality; chloride and bicarbonate concentrations and the serum pH will be normal.

In others, however, the biochemical picture of 'hypochloraemic alkalosis' is found. The elements of this are:

A raised serum pH: often in the range 7·50 to 7·55

A raised $pCO_2$, as part of the mechanism compensating the alkalosis

A raised plasma bicarbonate concentration—often in the range 30 to 45 mEq per litre—with a corresponding fall of plasma chloride.

Persistence of a paradoxically *acid* urine in the presence of alkalosis.

The mechanism of production of this state is not entirely clear: but the sequence is probably that excessive $K^+$ excretion involves an equivalent loss of body chloride ion. The chloride is withdrawn from the extracellular fluid and so potentially lowers the plasma chloride concentration; the 'anion gap' is then filled by $HCO_3^-$ from respiratory carbonic acid. The $H^+$ component enters cells to replace the K lost from them, and is buffered there by the cell proteins.

The alkalosis is *per se* of relatively little importance and will disappear when chloride ion is supplied in the diet. It is for this reason that potassium chloride and not potassium bicarbonate should be used for treatment of alkalosis accompanying $K^+$ depletion.

## Treatment of potassium depletion

Obviously, if there is a complex electrolyte disturbance, the replacement of K loss must be considered in the light of the whole disturbance. This applies particularly to gastro-intestinal catastrophes with large loss of gut secretions.

In pure K deficiency the best treatment for mild or moderate deficiency is to ensure that the patient takes an adequate amount of a high protein diet. In many frail, ill old people, and in those with surgical conditions where feeding by mouth is not feasible, the giving of oral K supplements will be necessary.

*Intravenous* potassium therapy should be reserved for severe potassium depletion with frank hypokalaemia, and under these circumstances:

1. Where life is threatened by the suddenness and severity of the K loss

2. When paralytic ileus has developed

3. Where frank skeletal muscle paralysis has appeared, especially if the respiratory muscles are involved.

*Practical details. Oral supplements.* All potassium salts in therapeutic use have unfortunately an unpleasant taste which is difficult to mask. For the supplementation of diuretic therapy, 20 to 30 mEq of K are needed daily. This is usually given as:

> Potassium chloride slow release tablet (Brit. Nat. Formulary)
> Tablet of 600 mg, i.e. 8 mEq of K and 8 mEq of Cl
> Dose: 1 table thrice daily (with meals to minimize the unpleasant taste); total daily dose gives 24 mEq of K.
> Or potassium chloride effervescent tablet (Brit. Nat. Formulary)
> Contains 12 mEq of K, 8 mEq of Cl and 4 mEq of $HCO_3$
> Dose: 1 tablet dissolved in water 2 or 3 times daily
> Total daily dose gives 24 to 36 mEq of K

For patients who cannot swallow tablets or tolerate their taste, two non-official (but expensive) solutions are:

'Kloref' (proprietary—no 'official' status) contains 6·7 mEq of K and 6·7 mEq of $Cl^-$ when put into solution. 'Katorin' (proprietary—no 'official' status) contains 14 mEq of K per 10 ml dose

Dose: 10 ml 2 or 3 times daily

Total daily dose gives 28 to 42 mEq of K

Oral potassium therapy is not without risk, especially in the presence of renal impairment, and the serum potassium level should be measured.

*Parenteral therapy.* Intravenous $K^+$ therapy requires skilled administration and monitoring since it carries a real risk of toxicity: if the infusion is administered too fast, blood $K^+$ concentrations reaching the myocardium can reach toxic or even fatal levels.

The two preparations available are:

1. Potassium chloride and sodium chloride injection (B.P.) Contains 0·3 per cent (w/v) KCl and 0·9 per cent NaCl, i.e. 40 mEq of K per litre and 150 mEq of Na per litre and 190 mEq of Cl per litre.

It is 'normal' with respect to sodium concentration, but 10 times concentrated in potassium. It is given without further dilution. The infusion rate absolutely must not exceed 5 ml per minute (equivalent to 12 mEq of K per hour). The serum $K^+$ concentration (and other electrolytes if the metabolic disturbance is complex) must be monitored every 2 hours.

2. Strong potassium chloride (B.P.)

This is prepared in ampoules of 10 ml containing 20 mEq of K and Cl. Its K concentration is five hundred times that of serum and is lethal if the solution is given intravenously undiluted.

If one ampoule (10 ml) is diluted into 500 ml of 0·9 per cent saline, and the mixture thoroughly shaken (the strong KCl solution has a high density and sinks to the bottom of the infusion vessel if proper shaking is not done), it is the same as the potassium chloride and sodium chloride solution (B.P.) described above.

The only advantage of the separate strong solution is that it allows variable K concentrations to be made up for use

by those experienced in parenteral therapy. Its use is
otherwise best avoided so that the risk of inadvertent
undiluted use does not arise.

# 16. Diabetes

Diabetes mellitus—'sugar diabetes'—is one of the enigmas of modern medicine. For many years it was very confidently believed to be a disease of carbohydrate metabolism pure and simple, its cardinal features being a raised blood sugar concentration and excretion of sugar in the urine: all other features of the disease were seen as 'complications'. While it is still true that hyperglycaemia and glycosuria are *sine qua non* for the diagnosis of diabetes and their correction is still the primary aim of treatment, this simple view of the nature of diabetes is now hotly contested. The pendulum has indeed swung so far in the other direction that one (minority) view sees diabetes as primarily a disease of small blood vessels, with the carbohydrate disorder as one of its results.

Although the ultimate basis of the disease may be obscure, the derangement of carbohydrate metabolism is incontestably due to an inadequate physiological effect of insulin, either because production of the hormone by the pancreatic islets is insufficient and the circulating insulin concentration consequently low, or because the tissues are less than normally sensitive to the hormone's metabolic effects (it promotes the transport of glucose across cell membranes, accelerates certain steps in the use of glucose as an energy source within cells, stimulates the formation in the liver of glycogen, a storage form of carbohydrate, and restrains the breakdown of fat in adipose tissue). It has been suggested by Vallance-Owen and his co-workers that tissue insensitivity is brought about by a circulating antagonist associated with serum albumin, but the the role of this substance is unproven. Randle and co-workers have suggested that in skeletal muscle insensitivity to insulin is due to the products of excessive fatty acid metabolism.

## Clinical features

It is usual to divide diabetes into two types. The *'juvenile'* or *'growth-onset' type* is characterized by: its severity—insulin therapy is, ultimately at any rate, always necessary; the prevalence of severe keto-acidosis; its abrupt onset, its occurrence in people of a normal or lean habitus and the development of weight loss as the disease takes hold. As the name implies. this type of diabetes begins in childhood or early adult life. Plasma insulin is present in low concentration or is absent.

The *'maturity onset' type* is milder, rarely shows ketosis and develops slowly. It occurs especially in obese, older people, and they show no weight loss as the disease evolves. The plasma insulin concentration is usually normal or raised; this is the type of diabetes in which the tissues are relatively insensitive to the hormone's action.

The vast majority of elderly diabetics belong to the maturity-onset group, but some patients with growth-onset, insulin-dependent diabetes survive into old age. The distinction between the two groups is in any case not sharp and maturity-onset diabetes can be temporarily changed by an acute infection or some severe general illness to show features of the juvenile type, keto-acidosis being the most important.

*Ways in which diabetes first presents in elderly people*
These are the common ways:

Glycosuria or a raised blood sugar level is disclosed as an incidental finding during the course of examination for some other disease; the patient is often completely free from diabetic symptoms.
The first symptoms are those of the complications: failing vision from cataract; intermittent claudication, gangrene of the toes or anginal pain from obliterative vascular disease; weakness and paraesthesiae from peripheral neuropathy.
Women commonly present with pruritus vulvae caused by a monilial infection.

Less common in old people are:
The classical symptoms of diabetes—excessive urine

flow, thirst, a large appetite, weight loss and lassitude. The polyuria is due to the fact that a large glucose excretion by the kidney will 'pull' water with it. To maintain water balance fluid intake must increase: in spite of great thirst, a proper balance is rarely achieved and some degree of dehydration usually results. Weight loss is due to combustion of the diabetic patient's own muscle and adipose tissue for energy production, because glucose, the prime, immediately available fuel, cannot be taken up or burnt in normal amounts.

Rare in old people is:
An acute onset in coma or precoma. This is only likely to occur in the elderly when moderately severe but unrecognized diabetes is suddenly transformed into the ketotic type by a severe infection or generalized illness. The condition develops over some hours or days and is never really abrupt as in hypoglycaemia, another cause of coma in diabetes. Abdominal pain and vomiting commonly occur and dehydration sets in rapidly, often with rapid, severe loss of visual acuity. The urine will contain large amounts of sugar and ketone bodies and the blood sugar usually exceeds 250 mg per 100 ml.

*Confirmation of the diagnosis.* The keystone of laboratory confirmation is the glucose tolerance test (GTT). The fasting blood sugar of a healthy person usually falls in the range 70 to 90 mg per 100 ml, but values up to 130 mg per 100 ml are normal for old people. Ordinary meals cause only a slight rise above the fasting value in health: insulin secretion in response to the meal stows glucose away almost as rapidly as it enters the circulation. For this reason a randomly timed blood sugar which exceeds 160 mg per 100 ml is very suggestive of diabetes. It is unwise to base so important a diagnosis on a single measurement and fuller confirmation is best obtained by the standard 50 g GTT, which deliberately stresses the body's capacity for handling carbohydrate. In this test the patient starves overnight; the following morning a 'baseline' sample is taken, the patient drinks 50 g of liquid glucose and then the blood sugar is measured at 30 minute intervals for $2\frac{1}{2}$ hours. The most important single BS value is that 2 hours after the glucose load. There are many ways of interpreting the GTT, but none is universally agreed as a standard. The following is a useful guide:

| | | |
|---|---|---|
| Severe diabetes (requiring insulin) | 2 hr BS | 200 mg per 100 ml |
| Definite diabetes | 2 hr BS | 140 to 200 mg per 100 ml |
| 'Borderline' diabetes | 2 hr BS | 120 to 140 mg per 100 ml |

*'Borderline' diabetes in old age.* The peak age incidence of freshly diagnosed diabetes is 60 to 70 years and as these patients have a life expectancy of about 9 years (65 per cent of the non-diabetic expectation), diabetes is predominantly a disease of elderly people.

The remarkable prevalence of diabetes in the elderly has been revealed by several community surveys. The 'Bedford Community Survey' of 1962 studied the prevalence of glycosuria in people on the electoral role of Bedford (known diabetics were excluded), in a sample of urine collected 60 to 90 minutes after a main meal. Glucose was found in 4 per cent of the whole group. The prevalence rose steadily with advancing age in men, reaching 8 per cent in men over 75, and was about half as high in elderly women. When these elderly patients with glycosuria were studied by GTT, slightly more than half the men over 69 years and 80 per cent of the women were diabetic as judged by the 2 hours BS value. An even more remarkable result was obtained when a random group of 570 people, stratified by age and sex, were studied by GTT (they were *not* selected for having glycosuria in the screening sample). In women aged 70, as many as 70 per cent had diabetic values as judged by the 2 hours BS level: but the great majority had only minor elevation above the 120 mg per 100 ml criterion. These were labelled 'borderline'. Professor Butterfield commented on the results thus:

'... if we subjected all the elderly grandfathers and grandmothers to glucose tolerance tests we would find that a very high proportion of apparently normal relatives of the normal population fulfilled current criteria for the diagnosis of diabetes.'

*The complications of diabetes.* Reference has already been

made to the argument surrounding blood vessel diseases in diabetes: are they really complications or are they an intrinsic part of the disease? The blood vessel lesions are of two types: a 'microangiopathy' affecting mainly capillaries, the primary lesion of which is a thickening and loss of structure in the basement membrane. There is evidence (not uncontested) that this change occurs before the development of a frankly diabetic disturbance of carbohydrate metabolism—a finding which speaks for the capillary lesions being an intrinsic part of the disease. Two organs are principally affected, the retina, where microaneurisms and haemorrhages develop in the fully flowered condition and cause severe loss of vision, especially when the macula is involved, and the kidney, where lesions in the glomerular tuft give rise to progressive renal impairment. These two conditions are usually late complications of the growth-onset type of diabetes, so they are uncommon in old people.

The second type of vascular complication involves larger vessels, especially the coronary and cerebral arteries and the vessels supplying the feet. Coronary involvement is of special importance, because it is the commonest cause of death from diabetes. The kind of lesions found in diabetes are not different in kind from the obliterative arteriosclerotic disease of non-diabetics—a ubiquitous disease and the main cause of death in the population at large, from middle age onwards.

The problem of prophylaxis is a very important one in relation to the vast numbers of old people with 'borderline diabetes'. Here the experience of the Bedford Community Survey is of interest. In a group of 'borderline' diabetics detected during the survey, treatment with tolbutamide for $8\frac{1}{2}$ years has shewn in the under 60's an advantage over placebo treated patients where cardiovascular morbidity was concerned. In the over 60's no such advantage emerged, perhaps because by chance a higher prevalence of heart disease in the drug-treated group on entry into the trial, as compared with the control group, obscured the result. At present there seems to be no positive evidence to justify the widespread prophylactic drug treatment of 'borderline' diabetes in old people without symptoms.

While it can be debated whether the vascular lesions of

diabetes are really 'complications', other disabilities are undoubtedly so. For the sake of completeness a table of the more important diabetic complications in late life is given below:

| Vascular: | (a) Obliterative disease of the large or medium arteries: coronary, cerebral, leg arteries |
| | (b) Lesions of capillaries |
| | retinopathy |
| | nephropathy |
| Ocular: | Cataract |
| | Vitreous opacities |
| | Glaucoma (usually secondary to retinopathy) |
| Nervous tissue: | Peripheral neuropathy |
| | Autonomic disturbance: |
| | overflow incontinence |
| | dysphagia |
| | diarrhoea |
| | impotence |
| Metabolic: | Non-ketotic hyperosmolar diabetic coma |
| | Diabetic coma (hyperglycaemia, keto-acidosis) |
| | Hypoglycaemic coma (effect of insulin or drugs) |
| Miscellaneous: | Special liability to infection of the skin and urinary tract, and to pulmonary tuberculosis. |

## Treatment of diabetes

There are four main methods of treating diabetes: insulin therapy; the use of oral hypoglycaemic drugs; restriction of carbohydrate in the diet and the reduction of weight if obesity is present. The principles are exactly the same for the old as for younger people. Every patient needs to be considered individually, but broad guidelines are:

| Severe | (1) 2 hour BS 200 mg per 100 ml or more (Heavy glycosuria and some degree of keto-acidosis often present) | Insulin will be needed |
|---|---|---|
| Moderate/ mild | (2) 2 hours BS 140 to 200 mg per 100 ml (Glycosuria, but ketosis mild or absent, symptoms usually present) | Insulin may or may not be necessary. If not, the hypo-glycaemic drugs will probably help. |
| Borderline | (3) 2 hour BS 120 to 140 mg per 100 ml (very often asymptomatic) | Decision on whether or not to treat will be determined by presence or absence of symptoms and complications. First line of treatment is carbohydrate restriction and weight reduction if obesity present. |

*Special aspects of treatment in the elderly*

*Insulin therapy.* The patient who has had a 'growth onset' diabetes for many years will probably already be experienced in the use of an insulin syringe but in those requiring insulin for the first time in later life, detailed instruction followed by checking of their capacity to administer the drug properly is needed. Confused old people usually cannot achieve this and insulin must then be given by a relative or District Nurse, or some other drug therapy used.

*Attention to foot hygiene.* The nails should be trimmed close and regularly by a chiropodist, the feet kept scrupulously clean and suitable footwear, i.e. shoes of soft material which avoid pinching or pressure on the toes, should be worn.

FURTHER READING

Malins, J. (1968) *Clinical Diabetes Mellitus*. Eyre and Spottiswoode: London.

Oakley, W.G., Pyke, D.A., & Taylor, K.W. (1968) *Clinical Diabetes and its Biochemical Basis*. Blackwell Scientific Publications: Oxford and Edinburgh.

Sharp, C.L., Butterfield, W.J.H. & Keen, H.A. (1974). *Proceedings of the Royal Society of Medicine*, **57**, 1964, 193–202. Diabetes Survey in Bedford, 1962.

# 17. Infections

Two common infections dwarf all others in importance in old people: pneumonia and urinary tract infection. Two others are worth mentioning because of their special features in old age: tuberculosis and subacute bacterial endocarditis.

## Pneumonia

Sir William Osler called pneumonia 'the old man's friend' because it often brought a welcome and relatively peaceful end to prolonged disablement and suffering. Although the advent of sulphonamide chemotherapy in 1936 and the antibiotics in the early 1940's provided powerful weapons against lung infections, pneumonia is still a serious matter in an old person. Even with the most potent chemotherapy expertly deployed, pneumonia continues to carry a 25 per cent mortality in old people. Why they should be so prone to pneumonia and why the death rate should be so high is not clear. The pat answer of 'general lowering of resistance to infection' in old age is hard to substantiate, as many other types of infection occur in the elderly, boils and wound infections for example, without the same overwhelming effect as pneumonia. The answer may lie in weakening of one or more of the lungs' specialized defences against bacterial invasion: these include coughing, ciliary action to promote upward streaming of mucus, immunoglobulin production by the respiratory epithelium and the phagocytic action of macrophages.

The causal agents are:

**Bacterial/viral**  *Streptococcus pneumoniae* (pneumococcus) and *influenza virus* account for about two thirds of fatal cases. The remainder are due to gram-negative organisms, the staphylococcus, *Mycoplasma pneumoniae* and viruses other than influenza, especially some rhino-viruses.

**Inhaled foreign material**   Vomit and food are the common offenders. Both are most likely to enter the lungs when consciousness is impaired and the cough reflex correspondingly depressed: in the early phase of stroke, after anaesthesia or in over-sedated patients are common circumstances. Impaired swallowing due to neuromuscular incoordination in the very old (presbyoesophagus) is another factor.

*Clinical features*

Although pneumococcus is a common causal organism, the classical picture of lobar pneumonia with an abrupt onset, fever and full-blown signs of lung consolidation is very much the exception.

The onset in old people is, typically, stealthy: the patient goes 'off colour', with lassitude, apathy and deterioration of mobility and general performance for two or three days, during which time there may be neither symptoms nor conspicuous signs to draw attention to a lung infection. The appearance of herpes simplex of the lips or pleuritic pain will strengthen suspicion, and eventually the triad of low fever, tachycardia and a raised respiratory rate will evolve (though fever can be absent throughout the illness). Local signs in the lungs in the early stage are often indefinite and consist of nothing more than patchy dullness and 'a few creps at the bases', but extensive lung signs may later appear with disconcerting suddenness.

This insidious onset is one of the factors in the high mortality of pneumonia: the disease has often taken a firm hold by the time that a cast-iron clinical diagnosis can be made.

Another general feature of pneumonia in the aged is the frequency with it presents as a confusional state: the possibility of an occult pulmonary infection should be considered in all old people who suddenly become confused.

## Influenzal pneumonia

Influenza 'A' is no more common in elderly people than in the population at large. Epidemics occur when the virus changes its antigenic properties and attacks a non-immune population, so the elderly are neither more nor less vulnerable in the antigenic sense than anyone else. True influenzal pneumonia only occurs in people who have the signs and symptoms of general invasion by the virus, and is therefore only likely to be seen during an epidemic. But the old are much more likely than the young to develop lung complications, and when they do the mortality is devastatingly high. Protection of old people by vaccination is advisable but offers nothing when the disease is already established.

## 'Terminal' pneumonia

'Terminal' pneumonia does not define a disease entity, but is applied to patients with severe debilitating disease who die from pneumonic infection. It is particularly in this situation that gram-negative bacteria or the staphylococcus tend to be responsible.

## Management

Management of pneumonia has three elements: chemotherapy, oxygen and good nursing.

Completely rational chemotherapy will involve prior identification of the causal organism, by direct smear and by culture of sputum. Unfortunately, many old people never produce sputum during pneumonia. Even if they do, and diagnostic facilities are quickly available, it is not justifiable to await treatment until the results are known. Strictly rational therapy which results in the demise of the patient gives comfort to none, and in many instances prompt therapy is required with no immediate bacteriological guidance. Treatment will for these reasons often be in two phases: first, treatment will start with the antibiotic likely to be effective on statistical grounds then, if the sputum smear or culture gives a clear indication of the pathogen responsible, a switch can be made to the most effective chemotherapeutic agent. Outside hospital wards many previously fit old people will be effectively treated by full oral doses of ampicillin. In hospital, where pneumonia is likely to occur in severely disabled people, the situation is more difficult, since a higher proportion of gram-negative and exotic pathogens is likely to be encountered. In these circumstances a broad spectrum antibiotic is indicated, for example, tetracycline in doses of 500 mg 6 hourly to begin with, reducing to half this dosage later. Whatever antibiotic is used, treatment should be continued for a minimum of seven days.

If the infection is overwhelmingly severe or oral therapy is impracticable, tetracycline intravenously to a daily total of 1000 mg is indicated.

*Oxygen therapy* is an essential part of treatment and is best given by a Ventimask delivering 28 per cent $O_2$ from a cylinder with a flow rate of 4 litres per minute, or by the Edinburgh type of face mask.

*Nursing care* is important for: (1) prevention of dehydration (many patients with pneumonia are stuporose or confused and drink little: they may quietly become grossly depleted of water); (2) special vigilance to prevent the development of pressure sores during the acute illness and (3) maintenance of nutrition and oral hygiene.

*Complications, course and prognosis*

The commonest immediate complication is congestive heart failure. Very often the patient also has ischaemic heart disease, and auricular fibrillation may make an unwelcome début during the course of pneumonia. A large, serous pleural effusion may also accumulate and require aspiration.

Pneumonia is slower to resolve in old people than in the young. Physical signs have usually cleared up in two or three weeks but X-ray shadowing often persists for up to six weeks. Persistence of signs and shadows for longer than this suggests an underlying lesion such as bronchial carcinoma, or bronchiectasis.

The high mortality has already been mentioned. The mental confusion precipitated by pneumonia does not always clear up when the infection subsides: return to the previous mental state may take several months or may never occur.

**Urinary tract infections**

The prevalence of urinary tract infections has been extensively studied in certain small groups of the population, notably school children and pregnant women. Despite the difficulties of obtaining specimens of urine uncontaminated by skin and vulval organisms, the results of different workers have agreed very closely.

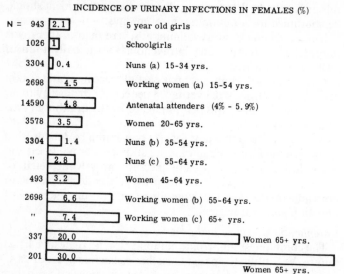

INCIDENCE OF URINARY INFECTIONS IN FEMALES (%)

| N = | 943 | 2.1 | 5 year old girls |
| | 1026 | 1 | Schoolgirls |
| | 3304 | 0.4 | Nuns (a) 15-34 yrs. |
| | 2698 | 4.5 | Working women (a) 15-54 yrs. |
| | 14590 | 4.8 | Antenatal attenders (4% - 5.9%) |
| | 3578 | 3.5 | Women 20-65 yrs. |
| | 3304 | 1.4 | Nuns (b) 35-54 yrs. |
| | " | 2.8 | Nuns (c) 55-64 yrs. |
| | 493 | 3.2 | Women 45-64 yrs. |
| | 2698 | 6.6 | Working women (b) 55-64 yrs. |
| | " | 7.4 | Working women (c) 65+ yrs. |
| | 337 | 20.0 | Women 65+ yrs. |
| | 201 | 30.0 | Women 65+ yrs. |

Fig. 17.1 Prevalence of urinary infection in females.

Figure 17.1 shows the trend in females. The prevalence of urinary infection rises from 1 to 2 per cent in female children to 3 to 6 per cent in women aged 15 to 64; it increased to 17 per cent in women in the general population over 65 and to yet higher levels for special populations such as those in Old People's Homes and geriatric hospitals. Comparable figures are not available for males, but it is likely that infection is less common in men than in women under 65. Thereafter the male prevalence rises and beyond the age of 70 urinary infection is as common in men as in women.

What are the causes and significance of this large increase in urinary tract infection in old age?

*Causes*

*Immobility* is an important aetiological factor in urinary tract infection. This is probably because immobility also causes constipation, which in turn may be associated with faecal soiling or incontinence. Contamination of the perineum and urethral orifice with coliform organisms leads to urinary infection in women. In addition, constipation and immobility can prevent complete emptying of the bladder.

*Residual urine* is another cause of infection. The normal bladder is emptied frequently and any organisms in the urine are evacuated before they have much time to multiply. Various types of neurogenic bladder will result in a large residual urine in both sexes (see p. 78) and prostatic hypertrophy is another common cause in men.

*Prostatectomy* also predisposes to bacteriuria, probably because the prostatic secretion contains an antibacterial substance which is lost when the gland is resected.

*Uterine prolapse* possibly predisposes to urinary infection. Surprizingly, however, bacteriuria does not relate to parity, nor to obstetric trauma at parturition, either from the use of instruments or perineal sutures.

*Senile vaginitis* (with its attendant changes in the epithelium of the urethra and trigone (see p. 74) has been implicated as a cause of bacteriuria but the evidence for this is inconclusive.

## Significance of bacteriuria

Although the aetiological factors mentioned have been established, it is not quite so easy to know what significance attaches to the bacteriuria. It is the local and systemic inflammatory reaction to bacteria rather than their mere presence which induces symptoms, as in the dysuria, incontinence and fever of acute cystitis. Treating the infection will, however, abolish these symptoms. Chronic bacteriuria on the other hand, while often associated with incontinence of urine or nocturnal frequency or precipitancy, is not likely to be the *cause* of these symptoms: it is more probable that whatever is causing the symptoms (e.g. bladder outlet obstruction due to prostate enlargement or a neurogenic bladder) leads to residual urine, and the chronic bacteriuria is a secondary phenomenon. In this case, treating the infection will not abolish the symptoms.

Although the urine may be sterilized by effective chemotherapy, reinfection by the same or another organism will in most cases occur within three or four months. In general, chronic bacteriuria seems to be, in old people, a relatively benign process which leads to neither renal failure nor hypertension (though it is regarded as much more sinister in younger age groups). For this reason, if treatment is followed by relapse, then further treatment is not usually pursued. However, a minority of elderly people with chronic bacteriuria do also suffer from pyelonephritis and while this will probably not respond to a short course of antibiotic or chemotherapy, the tendency to repeated recrudescences may be suppressed by more prolonged therapy.

*Diagnosis*

The diagnosis of urinary infection is now fairly standardized and is made on the basis of a bacterial count of a 'clean catch' specimen of urine when a count of 100 000 or more indicates the presence of infection. On a single specimen this is 80 per cent reliable. The bacterial count distinguishes between contaminants and infecting organisms, and since contaminants result from difficulty in collection, they will be found much more commonly in old people, particularly the immobile.

An alternative method of collection is by suprapubic aspiration of urine and this overcomes uncertainty as a result of contamination. However it excludes information on infection of the urethra. Suprapubic specimens are more likely to be successfully obtained in patients who cooperate well and who would therefore produce a more satisfactory mid-stream specimen in any case. In incontinent old people especially, it is not easy to achieve the degree of bladder distension necessary for this procedure to be carried out.

It is important that the specimen once obtained is sent to the laboratories at once and, if there is to be any delay, it should be put at once into a refrigerator. If kept at room temperature for half an hour organisms will multiply and the result may be in doubt.

The practical approach to urinary infection in the elderly is indicated in the accompanying flow diagram (Fig. 17.2).

Finally, it is worth stressing that a number of simple measures will help to prevent infection or its recurrence and

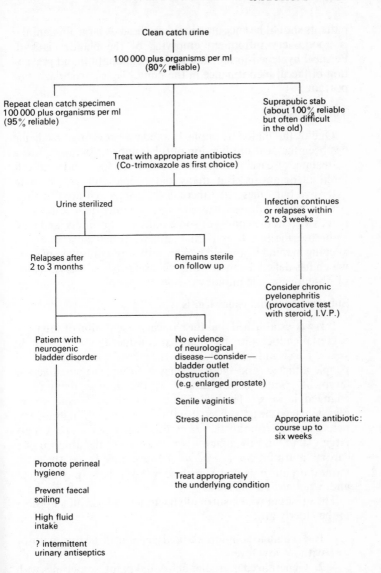

Fig. 17.2 The diagnosis of urinary infection.

patients should be encouraged to use these. A large fluid intake is good, very infrequent emptying of the bladder is bad. Perineal hygiene is important and the elimination and prevention of faecal incontinence in the immobile is particularly important.

## Tuberculosis

One of the major triumphs of modern preventive medicine has been the near-eradication of tuberculosis. As this is now a 'vanishing disease' it comes to mind much less readily in differential diagnosis. But many old people still survive with extensive but quiescent tuberculous lesions acquired in their youth when the disease was rife. Occasionally these lesions are reactivated in the course of some other minor illness, and tend to be overlooked. In particular miliary tuberculosis is worth keeping in mind in any old person with long-continued pyrexia which has defied diagnosis, and visceral tuberculosis is a cause of obscure chronic monocytosis in old people.

## Subacute bacterial endocarditis

It is well established that the clinical presentation of subacute bacterial endocarditis has changed considerably in the last 30 years. This is in large part due to the increasing number of old people afflicted, and the frequency with which their illness is 'atypical'. Some basic features of the disease remain unchanged, however. The infection commonly occurs on minimally damaged heart valves, usually the mitral, though incompetent and sclerotic aortic valves are affected to an increasingly large extent, and the diagnosis is insecure in the absence of a cardiac murmur. *Streptococcus viridans*, once by far the commonest organism is now run close by both the staphylococcus and *Streptococcus faecalis*.

The guises in which subacute bacterial endocarditis appears in the elderly are:

1. Weight loss, anorexia and general ill health, with or without low fever
2. Generalized muscular aches and pains, sometimes with transient joint pains—a symptom complex resembling 'polymyalgia rheumatica'

3. Progressively worsening heart failure without adequate explanation, often accompanied by rapidly increasing cardiac dilatation

4. Anaemia, with the morphological picture of anaemia of chronic disease (see p. 131) can dominate the picture

5. Persistent microscopic haematuria

6. Repeated embolism of the brain, central retinal artery or limbs

7. The geriatric common denominator—an acute confusional state

8. The classical text book picture of swinging fever, finger clubbing, splenomegaly and one or more Osler's nodes.

With such a bewildering large range of ways in which it can present, many of them with bizarre features, the possibility of subacute bacterial endocarditis will enter into the differential diagnosis of many old people's illnesses and the disease can only be detected with certainty by repeated blood cultures. The delay in diagnosis is usually several weeks and the mortality, even with optimal modern antibiotic therapy, is still very high in the long run.

# 18. Sensory Problems: Blindness and Deafness

## Blindness

Failing vision comes second in Shakespeare's list of the penalties of old age: 'sans teeth, sans eyes, sans taste, sans everything'. There are at present about 120 000 registered blind people in the United Kingdom, of whom 71 per cent are over 65. There are 12 000 new registrations per year.

Total or near total blindness in old people is always due to structural disease, either of the eye itself or of the nervous pathways concerned with vision, but a mild degree of visual impairment is an intrinsic aging effect, and so by definition is inevitable if the old person lives long enough.

## Age-determined changes in vision

These changes consist of:
**presbyopia**—reduced power of accommodation
**reduction of visual acuity**
**impaired dark adaptation**

*Accommodation* is the ability to form a sharp image of an object on the retina, over a range of distances from the eye and is achieved by 'fattening' the lens. The extent to which this can be done falls progressively throughout maturity and is closely correlated with age: at 20 years the lens has an accommodative range of about 10 dioptres (a dioptre is the optical strength of a lens with a focal length of 1 metre). This value falls to less than two dioptres at age 60 and is as low as 0·75 at 70 plus. Symptoms of accommodative stress, discomfort on attempting near vision, begin at 40 to 50 years, depending on race. This effect is probably due to the fact that the lens grows progressively throughout life: its equatorial diameter increases more than its thickness, so the radius of curvature becomes larger

These changes, plus decreasing elasticity of the lens substance cause long-sightedness in old people, and presbyopia.

*Visual acuity* is the equivalent of resolving power in a piece of optical equipment. It attains its best value at 20, then remains more or less constant till age 50, after which it slopes away gently until age 70; it then zooms steeply down, until as 80+ it is about one-quarter of the best value. However, at age 70, as many as 30 per cent of old people will still have full vision (with suitable correction of refraction) and at 80+ the figure is about 10 per cent. The changes responsible for this are not fully understood. *Senile miosis* is one factor. The pupil area is substantially smaller in old people, so the amount of light admitted to the eye, at a given illumination, is reduced, while the depth of focus is increased, exactly as in the 'stop' of a camera. Light-scattering and absorption in the lens and vitreous also contribute, but these two effects are not the whole explanation: some subtle central effect is probably also concerned.

While these intrinsic age changes cause some loss of vision, the remaining faculty is often perfectly adequate for the old person's limited needs, especially if illumination is good.

The common pathological causes of blindness acquired in old age are:

cataract
glaucoma
senile macular degeneration
diabetic and hypertensive retinopathy (the first much commoner)
optic tract lesions complicating stroke
cranial arteritis

*Clinical examination*

While detailed examination of visual function and eye disease is obviously a specialist matter, simple clinical methods give much information (though often neglected) and should include:

Examination of the external eye, for detection of corneal opacities, iritis, pupil changes, signs of previous operations

Crude tests of visual acuity—the ability to read print of

various sizes in a newspaper, or performance with Snellen's test card

Ophthalmoscopic examination—for detection of lens opacities as well as changes in 'the disc' and retinal bood vessels

Assessment of visual fields by confrontation.

*Cataract*

Cataract does not cause total blindness, but gives rise to mild or moderate visual loss of slow onset. Cataracts are due to local irregularities in the lens structure, either in its nucleus or cortex, which are opaque to light. They can be detected by focussing the ophthalmoscope beam on the lens rather than the retina and appear as greyish-black dots or lines, spidery figures or 'cuneiform' opacities. Accurate assessment requires examination with the narrow beam of a slit lamp. (The word 'cataract' derives rather obliquely from a Greek word for portcullis and presumably refers to the latticed appearance of opacities.)

As already mentioned, the lens continues to lay down new fibres throughout life: the most recent are on the outside, like the layers of an onion and optical discontinuities or 'disjunction stripes' accumulate throughout life, much as do the growth rings of a tree. Cataract is probably a genetically determined exaggeration and hastening of the normal aging changes in the lens and is, therefore, extremely common in old age. The special liability of diabetic and gouty patients and those receiving steroids is well-established.

Cataract is often bilateral, though there is frequently marked differences between the two sides. The disease does not cause total blindness, and rarely causes 'partial sightedness', but can cause severe loss of vision.

The management of cataract is a matter for the ophthalmologist. Patients with nuclear cataract often show increasing myopia and a change of glasses is often adequate treatment: dilatation of the pupil by homatropine (provided there is no risk of glaucoma) may also succeed.

Operative treatment consists of removal of the affected lens, Afterwards this has to be compensated by glasses, usually with an optical strength of about +10 dioptres plus a correction for astigmatism. These corrections cause spherical distortion and magnification of the image and the problems of the patient's adjustment, together with the increased risks of retinal detachment and glaucoma in the operated eye, make ophthalmic surgeons conservative in their approach to cataract in the aged, especially if 'the other eye' has adequate corrected vision.

### Glaucoma

The word is derived from the Latin for 'grey coloured'. This disease is due to a rise of intra-ocular pressure (normal pressure is 14 to 20 mm Hg) which, if prolonged can cause compression of the optic nerve head, and visual field defects.

Two distinct types are recognized:

1. *'Angle-closure glaucoma'* in which the aqueous humour cannot drain away, because the iris is jammed up against the filtration angle, closes Schlemm's canal and impedes the trabecular meshwork. The pressure rises to 45 to 60 mm. This type is predisposed to by a shallow anterior chamber (large lens) and a naturally acute angle.

Clinically, it presents:

*acutely* with severe pain in the eye, sometimes with vomiting, blurred vision and a cloudy oedematous cornea. The pupil is dilated, oval and non-reactive to light.

*subacutely*, i.e. with repeated minor prodromal attacks, in which there is pain in the eye, less severe than in the acute onset, blurring of vision and rainbow haloes on looking at lights.

*with an insidious onset* without ocular pain, haloes or blurring but with visual loss due to optic nerve compression.

This type of glaucoma may well be precipitated by ill-advised dilatation of a pupil with homatropine. Treatment of the acute attack is an emergency which should be dealt with in an ophthalmology ward and consists of intensive attempts to constrict the pupils with pilocarpine drops. If this fails, the carbonic anhydrase inhibitor acetazolamide can be given intramuscularly (500 mg, once) and if this in turn is unsuccessful, operation will be needed.

Chronic angle-closure glaucoma will need an iridectomy or drainage operation.

2. *'Open-angle glaucoma'* is due to impaired reabsorption of the aqueous humour and is of unknown cause. The patient usually presents because of visual impairment or the condition is discovered at routine examination through the detection of a 'cupped' disc, by an optician, ophthalmologist or even a general clinician. Treatment is again a specialist matter: if the patient has no material visual loss, medical measures for control of the intra-ocular pressure will be tried first. If the visual field loss is extensive and enlarging, a drainage operation will be needed.

### Senile macular degeneration

Since the macula is concerned with central vision, its 'degeneration', seen as whitish or grey mottling in the macular and perimacular region, often with some pigmentation, causes serious visual loss: the onset, fortunately, is fairly slow. The condition is probably hereditary. The only treatment possible is strong reading glasses and a magnifying glass for close work. Patients can often walk reasonably safely but are at a loss with work requiring detailed vision.

### Diabetic retinopathy

As with younger patients, retinopathy can be very severe in the presence of quite mild diabetes. It is revealed by the characteristic micro-aneurisms, haemorrhages and exudates: loss of vision ensues rapidly when the maculae are heavily affected.

### Visual field defects

A common defect in old people is a homonymous hemianopia complicating a cerebral thrombosis. The field of vision is lost to the midline in each eye, on the same side as the limb weakness, which is usually fairly severe. Provided the old person is capable of cooperating, the lesions can be detected by the simple confrontation test.

### Cranial arteritis

This is one of the few causes of acutely developing total blindness in old people and is to some extent preventable. The importance of early recognition and treatment has been stressed on page

## Effects of blindness on old people

A person who becomes blind in early life and grows old with the disability, will already have his life confidently organized, but blindness occurring out of the blue in an old person is a catastrophe which very often obliterates self-confidence and makes for total dependence on others. If there is a caring relative with whom the old person can live, much can be done in the way of social rehabilitation, but for those living alone complete self-care is rarely possible. Blindness is no bar to admission to Old People's Homes but the usual standard of competence in dressing, feeding and toilet is required, and many recently blinded old people will fall far short of this.

Learning to read Braille is beyond the capacity of most blind elderly, but the large better 'Moon' system is sometimes feasible. A recent innovation is the Talking Books Postal Service run by the British Talking Book Service for the Blind. Either the old person may apply direct or the Social Services can apply on his behalf (a special certificate from an ophthalmologist is needed before the service can be used).

### Legal aspects

The statutory definition of 'blind' under the National Assistance Act of 1948 is that the person is 'so blind as to be unable to perform any work for which eyesight is essential'. In reaching this definition (which can only be made by a registered ophthalmologist) all other physical or mental disabilities are disregarded. There are several qualifications to the definition: they are set out with form 'B.D. 8' which must be completed by the ophthalmologist. There is no compulsion to be 'registered', but only those on the Blind Register (which is kept by the Social Services Department) qualify for the few extra statutory benefits available. At present there is a small statutory increase in supplementary pension benefits for a blind person, but there is no separate 'Blind Pension'.

'Partial-sight' is defined so: '. . . illness or injury has caused defective vision of a substantial and permanently handicapping character. . . .' The persons are entitled to the welfare services for the blind provided by the Local Authority, but do not qualify for the Supplementary Benefit mentioned above. The relatives of a blind person may apply for the Attendance Allowance in the same way as for disablement from any cause.

## Hearing

One of the most obvious attributes of aging is an increasing difficulty in hearing. To what extent is this an age change and to what extent is it an age-associated disease change? The possible causes of impairment of hearing with age are many, for instance, primary degeneration of the organ of Corti with loss of epithelial nerve cells commencing in middle life. Changes have been reported in sensory cells of the cochlea, in both afferent and efferent nerve fibres, and changes in the spiral ganglion cells in the base of the cochlea. In addition a loss of elasticity in the basilar membrane of the cochlea and also in the eardrum have been reported.

Apart from these effects in the organ of hearing itself the blood supply of the neurosensory receptor may be impaired and both the auditory pathways and the temporal lobe of the brain may be affected by aging.

It seems clear, therefore, that age change in hearing may well be multifactorial in cause. Not only have several age and pathological changes been identified as possible causes but there are also several types of hearing loss occurring with advancing age.

'Presbyacusis' is a loss of pure tone hearing in the higher frequencies. This is an age related phenomenon.

Hearing may, however, be impaired because of these additional factors:

Tinnitus has been shown to increase in prevalence from 3 per cent in the second decade of life to 10 per cent in the sixth decade, though tinnitus is not necessarily associated with hearing loss.

Abnormal loudness perception. In about half of those patients who suffer from presbyacusis there is also hypersensitivity to very loud speech and an intensity level which would be acceptable to the normal person becomes unacceptable to the presbyacutic.

*Impairment of sound localization.* This may affect hearing by impairing the ability of the person to discriminate among the sounds heard in a noisy environment.

Simply identifying the loss of high frequency tones by audiometry carried out in a sound-proofed room will not, therefore necessarily give a good assessment of the hearing difficulty experienced by old people. In addition some tests involving the selection of one out of a number of sound signals will be required. Lip reading also may form a compensation for some hearing loss.

Different surveys have indicated different levels of hearing difficulty among the average aged population. The figure seems to lie somewhere between 12 and 30 per cent depending partly on the criteria used; in any event it is a sizeable proportion of the elderly population. For this reason assessment of the cause of hearing impairment is worthwhile in all elderly patients.

The first step is to exclude *wax* in the outer ear. This has been found in about one third of elderly patients who complain of deafness and sometimes its removal is all that is required to restore an acceptable level of hearing.

The second step is to provide an adequate electronic *hearing aid* and careful instruction in its use, together with follow-up support and encouragement. Hearing aids have many limitations, since increasing the volume of speech will not necessarily increase its intelligibility, and abnormal loudness perception may limit the degree of amplification which is acceptable. The use of two hearing aids (one in each ear) is better than one and the best results will be obtained in face-to-face conversation. The effect of a hearing aid in listening to what is being said at a distance is to pick up all the other extraneous sounds in the room. The result is akin to that of a tape recorder which has been placed to pick up group conversation and which seems particularly to magnify extraneous sounds such as door-banging and people coughing.

Although hearing trumpets seem clumsy they can be effective in face-to-face conversation.

One penalty of deafness is that it robs the sufferer of listening to radio and television programmes, and of conversation on the telephone. In each of these cases it is possible to provide special adaptors which may function with the patient's own

hearing aid. It is also useful to add a flashing light as a substitute for door-bells and other alarm signals.

Drugs have nothing to offer in the management of presbyacusis.

# 19. Nutrition

Impairment of nutrition may manifest itself either as *under-nutrition*, that it an insufficient intake of essential nutrients, or as overnutrition, that is *obesity*. Disorders of nutrition in either of these conditions may lead to disease. On the other hand they may be the result of disease.

In the elderly it is important to consider, first of all, whether there is any evidence that nutrition is impaired, secondly, what are the associated factors with individual nutrients, and thirdly, how nutrition may be improved or maintained in old people. The nutritional state can be assessed in three ways:

By measuring dietary intake

By measuring blood or tissue levels of the various nutrients

By looking for clinical evidence of subnutrition.

Only the third of these is likely to give firm evidence of subnutrition since both the dietary intake and blood and tissue levels may vary with age and as a result of associated diseases.

A very good definition of malnutrition is that proposed by Berry, namely: *'A disturbance of form or function due to lack or excess of one or more nutrients'*.

Before considering whether or not there is any malnutrition in the elderly a few known facts in relation to aging and dietary intake can be stated.

*Diet and longevity*

Well-known experiments with rats, comparing one group maintained on a restricted diet throughout their lives with another allowed to eat *ad lib* showed that those on the restricted diet had a longer life span, although they looked thin and less attractive. If the overfeeding was restricted to the period of growth it hastened maturity but shortened life. If, on the other hand, the animals were fed a restricted diet until maturity and thereafter were allowed to overfeed, the incidence of disease in old age seemed to be increased.

*Dietary surveys in old age*

The Department of Health and Social Security organized a survey of dietary intake and various aspects of nutrition among old people in several different and representative parts of the country. Altogether 879 people took part (425 males and 454 females). They kept diaries of the amount of food they had eaten; they underwent a clinical examination and analysis of blood levels and tissue levels of certain nutrients, and information about their social situation was taken into consideration. The most striking result of this survey was that only 3 per cent of the elderly population were regarded as malnourished. The daily intake of nutrients and energy is shown in Table 19.1 and if this is compared with the daily intake of energy and nutrients for elderly people recommended by the DHSS in 1969, the comparison shows the actual intake in almost all substances to be higher than the recommended intake (Table 19.1).

Table 19.1 Daily intake of nutrients and energy based on DHSS Survey of nutrition.

| | Recommended intake Men 75 + Women 75 + | | Actual intake (Women) Living alone | Living with family |
|---|---|---|---|---|
| Energy intake | | | | |
| (M cal) | 2100 | 1900 | 1890 | 1940 |
| (MJ) | 8.8 | 8.0 | 7·9 | 8·1 |
| Protein (g) | 53 | 48 | 62 | 62 |
| Fat (g) | | | 86 | 93 |
| CHO (g) | | | 232 | 228 |
| Calcium (mg) | 500 | 500 | 845 | 758 |
| Iron (mg) | 10 | 10 | 10.7 | 11.1 |
| Vitamin A (μg retinol equivalents) | 750 | 750 | 3560 (iu) | |
| Thiamine (mg) | 0.8 | 0.7 | 0.86 | |
| Riboflavine (mg) | 1.7 | 1.3 | 1.1 | not calculated |
| Nicotinic acid (mg equivalents) | 18 | 15 | 9.2 | not calculated |
| Ascorbic acid (mg) | 30 | 30 | 31 | |
| Vitamin D (μg cholecalciferol) | 2.5 | 2.5 | 71 (iu) | |

This large survey was of the population in general. Others have looked at more restricted groups of elderly people and by doing so have been able to demonstrate those who are particularly at risk as regards malnutrition. From these it appears that dietary intake diminishes only slightly with age in healthy old people, but it diminished very considerably in those suffering from disabling diseases. There are also considerable differences in the blood and tissue levels of certain nutrients in groups of people living in old peoples' homes or long stay hospital wards, as compared to the normal elderly population. This would seem to be due to increasing physical disability among the first two groups.

If we consider the individual nutrients, protein nutrition seems little affected by age.

*The B group vitamins* (thiamine, pyridoxine and nicotinic acid) show diminished blood levels in disabled old people which can be restored to normal by adequate supplementation. In the main, these low blood levels of B vitamins are not matched by clinical signs of subnutrition, but in a number of cases *angular stomatitis, cheilosis* (red, denuded, scaly epithelium in the line of closure of the lips) and a sodden appearance of the dorsum of the tongue, are associated with these deficiencies and can be reversed by supplementation. Angular stomatitis and tongue changes in particular are both multifactorial and may be caused by fungal infestation in the mouth, and indeed by the wearing of dentures.

*Ascorbic acid* (vitamin C). Blood levels of this vitamin again tend to be low in the disabled elderly, particularly those in hospital, but it is uncommon to find evidence of frank scurvy. Scurvy occurs most frequently in elderly men living alone.

*Vitamin $B_{12}$ and folic acid.* These vitamins are dealt with in more detail on page 127. Lower blood levels of both have been found in a small group of the elderly population, other than those suffering from anaemia, and again these are mainly people who are disabled or admitted to hospital.

*Vitamin A.* There is no evidence of vitamin A deficiency among old people in UK.

*Vitamin D.* Adequate vitamin D status requires both a sufficient intake and also exposure to sunlight, and this latter may be very important among elderly people in Great Britain. Lack of vitamin D leads to the disease osteomalacia and there is some evidence that osteomalacia is more common in the months January to June than July to December (p. 108).

## The assessment of nutrition

A simple assessment of an individual old person's diet may be made by finding out how many hot meals he has each week, and in addition how much milk he consumes and whether or not he eats fruit and green vegetables.

A survey carried out among the over 80's in Stockport indicated that only 60 per cent of the males, and 48 per cent of the females had one hot meal each day, and that 17 per cent of the males and 23 per cent of the females had two or less hot meals each week. The general practitioner or the health visitor can easily make some assessment of nutritional status from answers to these simple questions.

### 'At risk' groups

It seems clear from what has been written above that, in general, the elderly population of Great Britain is adequately nourished but there is a group of old people who have an unsatisfactory dietary intake, and low blood and tissue levels of nutrients, although these are not always matched by clinical signs of malnutrition. It is these, 'At Risk' groups who should be identified and for whom doctors should take action to improve their diet. They include the following:

1. Those who are socially isolated; particularly very old men living alone
2. Those with physical disease, because this makes it difficult for food to be handled or swallowed, and because immobility tends to diminish appetite
3. Those with sensory impairment (sight, hearing, taste and smell) who may have diminished appetite, and who also for these reasons may fall into the socially isolated group
4. The bereaved; the period of grieving is associated with loss of appetite. If it lasts for an appreciable time it may tip the balance in a very old person who is already on the nutritional borderline
5. Those suffering from mental disease, in particular depression.

*Management*

Every old person should have at least five hot meals a week, and anyone who is unable to prepare these adequately for himself should be supplied with Meals on Wheels or preferably attend a luncheon club or a social day centre (transport will almost certainly be required). If Meals on Wheels are necessary as the chief form of nutrition it is essential that they be provided five days a week. Anything less than this, while it may be good supplementation to a diet already adequate, or may add variety to the monotonous diet of the housebound, is not sufficient of itself to maintain adequate nutrition.

*Vitamin supplementation.* The question of vitamin supplementation is a difficult one. While there is no doubt that small groups of old people have inadequate vitamin intake there does not seem to be any justification for the wholesale vitamin supplementation of old peoples' diets. Evidence of diseases such as osteomalacia and scurvy clearly indicates the need for supplementation. There is also a good case to be made out for vitamin supplementation of the 'at risk' groups, defined above, together with long stay patients in hospital and disabled people in old peoples homes or living alone. This should be with water soluble vitamins (B group and C) and vitamin D.

*Energy.* Nutritional needs are directly related to the expenditure of energy. In old age this is diminished in a number of ways. Increased disability leads to decreased exercise; retirement also causes diminished energy expenditure. However, in modern society automation has removed the significant energy expenditure from very many forms of occupation. Public and private transport and a general half-heartedness towards playing energy-expending games on the part of much of the population means that the differences between the energy expenditure of the old and the rest of the population are probably less now than in the past.

## Obesity

Changes in the disposition of fat stores seems to occur in human beings as they age, with movement of fat from subcutaneous tissues to deep tissues, and from the limbs to the trunk.

Generally speaking obese people do not survive into old age. Those who do are often found to have a lower calorie intake than the non-obese. They do not burn up their fat stores however, because they are economical of physical effort and indeed, if disabled, they may be immobile. In such circumstances weight reduction by calorie restriction is a long drawn out process, requiring strong motivation. Without such motivation on the part of the patient, success is unlikely to be achieved.

## FURTHER READING

Durnin, J.V.G.A. (1973) Nutrition. In *Textbook of Geriatric Medicine and Gerontology*, p. 384, ed. Brocklehurst, J.C.

# 20. Periphero-vascular and Musculo-skeletal Disorders

In this chapter it is intended to deal with a number of clinical conditions which, while common or with their maximal incidence in advanced age, nevertheless are well recognized by physicians and surgeons and well dealt with in textbooks of medicine and surgery. It is not intended, therefore, to deal with them extensively, but simply to bring out those points which are of particular importance in old age.

## Peripheral arterial disease

It is apparent that atherosclerosis is the basic pathological condition underlying a great deal of morbidity in the elderly and one of its important effects is to produce the *ischaemic foot*. This may present clinically in one of three ways:

Pain alone: either intermittent claudication occurring in the calf or rest pain in the foot, often confined to the heel, and often occurring during the night

Pre-gangrene: discolouration of part of the extremity of the foot, usually but not always associated with pain

Gangrene: discolouration associated with coldness and usually with pain.

Both gangrene and pre-gangrene may be associated with bacterial infection particularly around the nail or between the toes.

### Management

Clinical assessment of all peripheral pulses should be a routine part of every physical examination in old people and in peripheral arterial disease most careful note must be taken of the presence and nature of the arterial pulses in the groin and the popliteal fossa as well as the posterior tibial, and the dorsalis pedis. Additional information about the peripheral circulation can be obtained by an aortogram or an arteriogram but these should only be carried out if it is intended to proceed to vascular surgery should an operable arterial obstruction be discovered (and of course these procedures would never be done in a patient with gangrene).

There are two specific methods of approach to peripheral vascular disease in old people, firstly, to improve the collateral circulation, and secondly, arterial surgery (either endarterectomy or replacement by graft or prosthesis of an obstructed part of the artery). Unfortunately, atherosclerosis is generally so widespread, often with several major areas of obstruction that neither of these approaches is helpful.

If pain only is present then an attempt should be made to improve the collateral circulation by increasing periods of daily exercise, for instance on a treadle, and by clinical trial of a vasodilator. The latter includes papaverine, nicotinamide, priscoline ('Priscol') and more recently introduced substances such as cyclandelate ('Cyclospasmol') and naftidrofuryl ('Praxilene'). If any of these is found to relieve the pain then it may be continued with, but if not, then the clinical trial should not extend beyond three or four weeks. In pregangrene the use of intra-arterial 'Priscol' has been recommended in the past and there is now some evidence that intravenous 'Praxilene' has some effect. This is also the condition in which arterial surgery should be considered. General measures include rest and the prevention of superadded infection.

In patients who suffer from gangrene early consultation with a surgeon is important, and months of suffering may be short-circuited by an appropriate amputation.

Diabetes is a common underlying cause of peripheral atherosclerosis and must always be looked for.

### Venous thrombosis

Superficial thrombophlebitis manifests itself as redness and pain limited to part of the calf, and the affected vein is tender. It is usually treated by firm binding of the leg with a crepe bandage, analgesics and restricted activity but not complete rest. Recurrent episodes of superficial thrombophlebitis (thrombophlebitis migrans) are sometimes an early sign of an unsuspected carcinoma.

*Deep vein thrombosis*

This is particularly important in the elderly, especially in those who are immobilized (e.g. as a result of a stroke) or those undergoing pelvis surgery or surgery of the hip joint. Its especial importance lies in the fact that it frequently leads to pulmonary embolism, a not uncommon cause of death in old people. The other long-term complication of deep venous thrombosis may be peripheral stasis with the production of leg ulcers.

Deep vein thrombosis occurs insidiously and is often un-diagnosed until embolism occurs, though swelling and tender-ness of the calf, oedema of the affected foot and pain on dorsiflexion of the affected foot (Homans' sign) can often be detected if the legs are examined routinely. Some geriatricians advocate the routine scanning of the legs of patients who are at risk, to detect thrombosis before these clinical signs de-velop. The scanning is by a Geiger counter after the patient has taken fibrinogen labelled with radioactive iodine [125]I. This becomes incorporated into the thrombus.

Prevention is also important. All old people lying in bed should be encouraged to keep their legs moving. Some ortho-paedic surgeons use routine anticoagulants in patients under-going operation for fracture of the neck of the femur.

Treatment is by elevation of the limb and the early use of anticoagulants (care being taken to consider contraindications, which are many in old people). Phenylbutazone is the drug of choice in managing the pain of thrombophlebitis and in addi-tion its anti-inflammatory activity may contribute to resolu-tion of thrombus.

Various methods of preventing pulmonary embolus in patients with deep vein thrombosis have been used, including the implantation of devices into the inferior vena cava to entrap emboli at that level: none of these has achieved general acceptance in the elderly. An alternative to anticoagulants, where they are contraindicated, is the use of Dextran 70 ('Macrodex') which diminishes platelet adhesiveness and thus reduces coagulability.

## Chronic leg ulcers

Chronic leg ulcers can be most intractable in elderly people.

They occur in the lower third of the calf or around the ankle, may be single or multiple, painful or asymptomatic, and are associated generally with venous stasis either following deep vein thrombosis or in association with immobility and postural oedema of the legs. Management involves treatment of the superficial infection. Topical treatment is usually adequate, and systemic antibiotics are only indicated if there is an appreciable surrounding area of cellulitis. Chronic leg ulcers will usually heal with combination of bed rest, elevation of the limb and non weight-bearing active exercises. The healing process is slow and care must be taken to avoid other attendant risks of a period of immobility and bed rest. Daily physiotherapy is essential. Unfortunately, many leg ulcers relapse either as a result of minor trauma or because of recurring postural oedema in patients who remain chairfast. Elastic stockings should therefore be provided as soon as the ulcers have healed. Other methods of management which have been advocated are peripheral vasodilators, the administration of zinc sulphate by mouth and plastic surgery but results with these methods are generally disappointing.

### Osteo-arthrosis

Age associated change in synovial joints is extremely common even from early adult life and these changes are similar to those seen in osteo-arthrosis. It is not at all clear to what extent they are pathological and to what extent they are simply due to wear and tear with advancing age. Changes include unevenness of the articular surface, fibrillation and formation of clefts and fissures in the cartilage matrix. Erosion of hyaline cartilage causes eburnation of the bone and cyst formation in the subchondal marrow spaces. Such changes may be regarded as pathological when they are associated with additional factors which add to the trauma and stress experienced particularly by the large weight-bearing joints, as is the case in *secondary osteo-arthrosis*. Here one or more joints are affected, usually in an asymmetrical manner, often with considerable deformity and pain. The osteo-arthrosis may be secondary to obesity, previous joint diseases (e.g. Perthés), previous fracture and occupational trauma as in footballers, coal miners, dockers and furniture removers.

Secondary osteo-arthrosis is to be distinguished from the syndrome described by Kellgren and Moore as *primary generalised osteo-arthrosis*. The latter occurs in postmenopausal women, producing a symmetrical arthrosis affecting particularly the distal interphalangeal joints and first carpometacarpal joints, but also affecting all other joints including the apophyseal joints of the spine. It may have a subacute onset but in the rest of its course is a relatively benign condition and is characterized by Heberden's nodes.

## Rheumatoid arthritis

*Rheumatoid arthritis* can start acutely in advanced old age or else patients may grow old with it in a 'burnt out' form from earlier life. The acute form is often atypical of the disease in younger patients. It has a 'galloping' course affecting particularly the larger joints in the early stages. In about 25 per cent of acute cases in old age there is full recovery within 3 to 18 months.

The co-existence of chronic rheumatoid arthritis and osteoarthrosis sometimes poses diagnostic difficulties in the elderly. Rheumatoid involvement in the hands is generally in the proximal interphalangeal joints (as well as the metacarpophalangeal and wrist joints), whereas osteo-arthrosis affects the distal interphalangeal joints. The 'Bouchard node' may be a source of error: it represents a noninflammatory degenerative arthrosis affecting the proximal interphalangeal joints.

*A monarticular arthritis* (senile monarticular arthritis) has also been described and sheep-cell-negative acute polyarthritis is also a relatively common nonspecific joint disorder of the elderly which may last for a number of weeks with a painful and disabling rheumatoid appearance, and then clear up without trace. It is clear that further research is needed to clarify the classification of these various joint disorders in the elderly.

*Pseudo-gout* (or 'pyro-phosphate arthropathy') occurs in old age, attacking the large synovial joints. It is diagnosed by X-ray evidence of calcification of the articular cartilage (most commonly seen in the meniscus of the knee) and associated with presence of calcium pyrophosphate dihydrate crystals in the joint fluid. Aspiration of the affected joint will often cut short the attack.

## Back pain

Two age associated processes, osteoporosis and osteo-arthrosis may present as pain in the back and since these are so common it is important that patients presenting with this symptom should be considered for other possible causes. The differential diagnosis of back pain in old age includes, in addition to osteo-arthrosis and osteoporosis; osteomalacia, Paget's disease, metastatic carcinoma, prolapsed intravertebral disc and multiple myeloma.

# Part Four: Services for the Elderly

# 21. Geriatric Services

The Geriatric Service is an important part of the National Health Service in Great Britain. It is hospital based and organized by consultant geriatricians. The geriatric service is based on a geographical area which usually corresponds to the health service district. This may have a population of between 100 000 and 500 000 people altogether, of whom in most areas 14 to 15 per cent will be aged 65 and over (although this figure will be very much higher in retirement areas). The practice of geriatric medicine is based on the practice of general medicine but in many ways the method of organizing the work is more akin to that of the psychiatrist and paediatrician than to the general physician. The latter spends most of his day in consultation with individual patients to diagnose and advise about the treatment of acute episodes of disease: the geriatrician provides a service for an area which involves not only the management of individual ill patients but also the organization of a rehabilitation team, long term care, a day hospital, some form of ascertainment of unreported illness and maintenence of a close liaison with community services including voluntary services.

## Definition

It is not easy to produce a definition of geriatric medicine which would be acceptable to all geriatricians. It is basically a system of care rather than an age-related specialty but in some areas it is practised as an age-related specialty based on the lower age limit of 70 or 75 years. Perhaps the best definition is that of the British Geriatrics Society which is simple yet comprehensive:

> Geriatrics is the branch of general medicine concerned with the clinical, preventative, remedial and social aspects of illness in the elderly.

**Structure**

The geriatric service may be wholly or partly based in a district general hospital or part in a smaller hospital (now to be called a community hospital). The geriatrician usually organizes the beds in his care to provide a system of progressive patient care and involving stages of acute treatment, rehabilitation, continuing care in hospital and day hospital care.

*Acute geriatric wards*

These wards are situated in a district general hospital and to them come most patients on their first admission to the geriatric department. Here the initial investigation, treatment and assessment is carried out with the use of whatever ancillary services are required so that a complete series of diagnoses may be made, appropriate medical treatment instigated, and the patient's future social care considered. The method of working is much the same as in any other acute hospital ward and the length of stay should ideally be two to three weeks. From here the larger number of patients will go home or to an old people's home. Some will die and others will proceed to rehabilitation.

*Rehabilitation wards*

Rehabilitation wards are generally situated in the district general hospital—very often in association with the day hospital so that the patients may go to the day hospital for their treatment in the day time, returning to the wards in the later afternoon. Patients are generally transferred to the rehabilitation ward from the acute geriatric ward. Others may be transferred directly from medical, surgical and orthopaedic wards. Rehabilitation is mainly *the physical treatment of disability which is carried out with an expectation of improvement and in which the aim is to make the patient sufficiently independent to be able to live at home or in an old person's home.* Patients requiring rehabilitation are predominantly those suffering from stroke, Parkinsonism and arthritis in its various forms, together with patients recovering from fractures of the femur. However the whole spectrum of disabling disease will be dealt with here. The average length of stay is 8 to 12 weeks. At the end of that time the larger number of patients will return to their own homes or old people's homes. Some will have died and a small number will remain so disabled that they are unable to be discharged from hospital. These will then move to the third system of care—continuing care or long term care.

*Long term care*

Long term care beds may be situated in the district general hospital and also in other more peripheral hospitals: there are obvious advantages, particularly in rural areas, for patients requiring continuing hospital care to be able to live in a hospital near to their former home. Long term care wards are different in their purpose from other types of hospital wards. Patients are there because they require nursing and in most cases they are there for the remainder of their lives. The average length of stay is between two and three years.

This, therefore, is the patient's home and every effort must be directed to making it as homely as possible, free from discipline, where patients have every opportunity to do as they please. Although most students will associate hospital care only with acute wards, in fact the larger number of beds in the National Health Service are for long term and not acute care. Unfortunately few purpose-built long term care units exist in Great Britain; almost all of those used for geriatric long term care have been built for other purposes: infectious disease hospitals, tuberculosis sanitoria, workhouse infirmaries, general hospital wards, private houses, offices etc. This lack of purpose-building imposes a great handicap.

Ideally each patient should have his own bedroom and the wards should consist of a complex of lounge, dining room, recreation room, art studio and garden. The majority of long term geriatric patients can be mobile in wheelchairs and it is only in the last few weeks of an average stay of two to three years that they will be bedfast. Congenial and stimulating activities should be provided and every effort made to give some shape to the patients' week so that one day is not the same as every other day and one week the same as every other week. Everyone needs something to look forward to, day by day, and this applies more and not less to elderly people who have to live out their lives in a hospital. Great success has attended the provision of properly staffed and equipped classes in arts (including painting and modelling), crafts, musical activities and so on. These can be most conveniently provided by setting up adult education classes under the auspices of the Adult Education Department of the Local Authority within the hospital itself.

Patients should have as much freedom as possible. Volunteers may be recruited to act as visitor; both relatives and volunteers should be encouraged to take the long term patients out for a few hours' run in a car and visit private houses from time to time. Where possible arrangements should also be made for the patients to transfer to a seaside or country setting for a week or two during the year, as a holiday.

Figure 21.1 indicates the progression of patients through one geriatric department which is probably typical of most. It must be realized that only about 10 per cent of patients admitted to

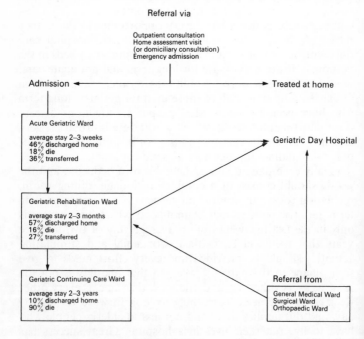

Fig. 21.1 The structure of geriatric care.

the geriatric unit end up by becoming long term patients, but since this group has such a disproportionately long period of bed occupancy, relatively larger numbers of long term beds are needed.

*Holiday admissions*

Most geriatric departments admit patients who are being nursed at home by their relatives on a short term pre-arranged admission to allow the relatives to have a holiday. Care of a disabled old person at home, particularly if there is some mental impairment, is a demanding and unremitting responsibility. Unless those who carry it out can obtain relief from time to time it is likely that the situation will eventually break down and long term care be sought for the old person. Holiday admission is a method of trying to prevent this breakdown.

## The geriatric day hospital

The day hospital is an extension of progressive care, beyond the period of in-patient treatment. It allows the patient to have the benefit of hospital investigation and treatment whilst still able to live at home at night and over the weekend. It is thus, both an advantage to patients, and economic of staff. Geriatric patients attend the day hospital for four main reasons:
1. Rehabilitation
2. Maintenance treatment
3. Social care
4. Medical and nursing investigation and treatment.

Patients with the same diagnosis may attend for any of these different purposes and it is extremely important that the geriatrician and all his staff should be aware of the reasons why each patient is attending. The principal diagnosis itself will not necessarily give an indication of this.

*Rehabilitation*

Rehabilitation may continue after the patient leaves hospital (perhaps allowing him to leave earlier than might otherwise be the case), or may be carried out entirely on a Day Hospital basis without previous admission. Rehabilitation envisages improvement and once improvement ceases and the patient reaches the maximum degree of independence then rehabilitation should also be withdrawn. At this stage it is necessary to decide whether the patient's situation and motivation are sufficient for him to maintain the degree of independence which he has reached or whether he requires frequent and regular supervision from the hospital to help him to maintain this. In this case he requires maintenance treatment.

### Maintenance treatment

This is in effect, the provision of physical treatment one day a week to retain the gains that have already been obtained. Maintenance treatment may continue indefinitely.

### Social care

Social care may be provided in the Day Hospital for patients whose disabilities are so great that they need constant nursing assistance. Such patients attend for two reasons:

1. So that they may be cared for each day while relatives go out to work

or

2. So that they may be cared for one day a week to give their relatives a break and to allow the patient an opportunity of socialising and meeting other people.

Care of this type for patients who are not disabled and do not require nursing assistance would normally be provided at a day centre which is run not by the hospital service but by the local authority.

### Medical and nursing procedures

Many procedures can be carried out in a day hospital which require a period of observation over several hours, perhaps repeated on several days, e.g. in the elucidation of incontinence, stabilization of drug therapy, or procedures which can be carried out in a single visit such as a glucose tolerance test. Most day hospitals provide a large number of enemas and also a number of baths.

### Management

The day hospital should be managed in a dynamic way: patients should attend for a limited period of time, being discharged whenever possible. Since discharge often means going back to isolation after having enjoyed a period of socialization, it is often helpful to transfer the patients who no longer need day hospital care, to a day centre. Day centres provide social care and indeed many of them provide baths, hairdressing, laundry, chiropody and other services but they do not have the medical, nursing and therapeutic staff as does the day hospital. They are usually managed by the Social Services Department of the local authority.

The medical management of a day hospital is very similar to that of a hospital ward. Day-to-day contact between junior medical staff and patient is essential and there should be a weekly round or case conference with the consultant geriatrician.

## Relatives' clinics

A number of geriatric departments are now developing 'relatives' clinics' or 'relatives' conferences' so that the relatives of old people who are geriatric patients may have an opportunity of meeting together to discuss their common problems and meeting with members of the staff to receive instruction and advice. Such conferences provide a form of group therapy for the often hard pressed relatives (who sometimes feel unjustifiable guilt at being unable to cope) allowing them to obtain confidence by knowing that their problems are not unique. The conference also allows demonstration of ways of managing the common problems of disabled old people.

## The psychiatry of old age

The psychiatry of old age is gradually emerging as a special branch of psychiatry analogous with child psychiatry. The psycho-geriatrician (as he is sometimes called) is a psychiatrist with responsibility for the complete management of the whole range of psychiatric problems in old age. He is likely to have a complement of both acute and long term care beds and a day hospital. Very often the acute ward is jointly staffed with the geriatrician (and called a Psycho-geriatric Assessment Ward). The intention is, as far as possible, to admit all confused old people coming into hospital into this ward, to allow a comprehensive and clear diagnosis to be made of the cause of confusion, and for this to be managed as far as possible within the ward. If care extending beyond four weeks or so is needed then transfer to an appropriate longer term setting must be agreed at case conferences held jointly between the psychiatrist, the geriatrician and the social worker. In general, patients needing long term care will be dealt with as follows:

1. Those suffering from affective disorders or from the chronic brain syndrome with associated behavioural problems will be looked after by the psycho-geriatrician.

2. Those with the chronic brain syndrome who are ambulant and do not provide behavioural problems such as persistant wandering, aggression or antisocial activity will be looked after by the Social Services Department in its residential home

3. Those suffering from the chronic brain syndrome but whose problems are basically those of physical incapacity will be looked after by the geriatrician.

It is assumed that within four weeks most patients with acute confusional states will be diagnosed and successfully treated.

The Psycho-geriatric Day Hospital should be separate from, although it can adjoin, the Geriatric Day Hospital. Its primary function is to look after old people suffering from the chronic brain syndrome while their relatives work, or to provide their relatives with some freedom. At the same time it should provide a suitable group atmosphere for the treatment of these patients.

## The ascertainment of unreported illness

It is well known that old people frequently suffer from an illness which produces apathy, lethargy, pain, giddiness, falling, urinary problems and others, without ever seeking treatment for these by reporting them to their doctor. The reason is that they mistakenly believe that such symptoms are due to aging rather than disease, and that nothing can be done about them. For this reason there has been much thought and research into the question of whether there is a need to set up a special service to ascertain unreported illness in old people. An early research project designed to answer this question was carried out by Williamson in Edinburgh (1964). Williamson and his colleagues examined the old people in a series of general practices, thereby obtaining an adequate sample of the total elderly population of Edinburgh. The patients were examined in detail both physically and psychiatrically and all their illnesses were documented. The research workers then went to the general practices to discover how much of the illness that was documented by them was known to the general practitioner because the patient had reported it. These findings may be discussed under two headings: first *diseases of the major systems*. Figure 21.2 shows the prevalence of such

INCIDENCE OF DISEASE IN THE ELDERLY

(Williamson et al 1964)

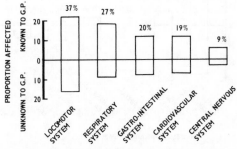

Fig. 21.2 The assessment of unreported illness (1).

disorders, indicating above the line the proportion of this illness known to the general practitioners and below the line the proportion which was not known to them. It is immediately apparent that there is a very great deal of morbidity among the elderly. Disease of the musculo-skeletal system affecting 37 per cent of the over 65's is not surprising since disc degeneration and degenerative arthrosis are the common accompaniments of aging. However a 27 per cent prevalence of respiratory disease in old people of Edinburgh is a more surprising figure, and it is matched by disease of the gastrointestinal system in 20 per cent, of the central nervous system in 9 per cent and of the cardiovascular system in 19 per cent. In most cases, apart from disease of the musculo-skeletal system, the doctor was aware of the larger proportion of this illness because no doubt he had been involved in investigating it in the past and in treating its acute episodes. Moreover it is likely that the considerable amount of disease of the musculo-skeletal system about which he is unaware and the rather smaller amount of disease of the other systems that he is unaware of, include much that is not accessible to therapy. On the basis of these figures, therefore, it is doubtful whether a case can be made out for the deployment of staff on extensive (and expensive) medical examinations of old people.

Figure 21.3 shows a rather different series of illnesses. These

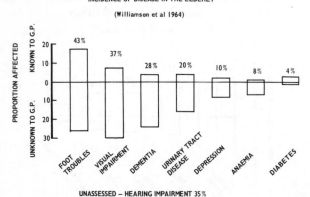

INCIDENCE OF DISEASE IN THE ELDERLY

(Williamson et al 1964)

UNASSESSED – HEARING IMPAIRMENT 35%

Fig. 21.3  The assessment of unreported illness (2).

are *more discrete disabilities and more easily susceptible to treatment*. They are disabilities which may progress, and pre-dispose to accidents and isolation. They include foot disorders in 43 per cent, visual disorders in 37 per cent, urinary disorders in 20 per cent, dementia in 28 per cent, depression in 10 per cent, anaemia in 8 per cent and hearing disorders in 35 per cent. Figure 21.3 indicates that most of these will be unknown to the doctor because they have not been reported to him and that in most cases the conditions are treatable. Certainly in the case of anaemia, depression, many visual disorders, hearing impairment, and many of the urinary troubles, specific therapy is available. In the case of dementia (where the figure is ex-tremely high probably because it includes mild, as well as moderate and severe dementia) treatment is unlikely to be very profitable. However, a good deal of care and support can be offered to the relatives through day care and intermittent admission of the patient to an Old Person's Home.

There would seem, therefore, to be every reason to ascertain disabilities of this type. Moreover they may be looked for by someone whose training has not been as extensive as a doctor's. Many general practitioners have Health Vistors attached to their practices, who can be equipped and trained to test vision and hearing, look for foot troubles, and oedema, consider the possibilities of depression and dementia and take a sample of blood and urine. The practice Health Visitor armed with a complete list of the over 70's in the practice is in a unique position to offer this service as well as affording advice to these old people on diet, social services and other aspects of health maintenance.

It seems likely that this pattern of the ascertainment of unreported illness is the one which will be followed in the future.

## FURTHER READING

Brocklehurst, J.C. (Ed.) (1975) *Geriatric Care in Advanced Societies*. Lancaster: M.T.P.

# 22. Social Services

## Historical background

There has been some kind of statutory social service in Great Britain since 1601, when the Poor Relief Act set the responsibility for the poor and disabled squarely on the shoulders of the local parish. It was laid down that the able-bodied should work, children should be bound apprentice and the halt, the lame, the impotent and the blind should be given relief. Care of the old has ridden on the back of care of the disabled ever since.

This system worked reasonably well for more than 200 years, until 1834, when a Board of Guardians was set up to supervise conditions, and adopted the principle of 'less eligibility' which really meant that 'the workhouse' was to be made sufficiently less pleasant than life outside, as to discourage people from entering it, and so it was. Modern protests against state support of 'layabouts' are perhaps distant echoes of the same attitude expressed in the Commissioners' report of 1834, which, while recognizing that the 'aged poor of good conduct' had a claim to special treatment, said about the aged poor of bad conduct: 'For the old men and women of this kind the general mixed workhouse with its stigma of pauperism, its dull routine, its exaction of such work as its inmates can perform, and its deterrent regulations seems a fitting place in which to end a mis-spent life'. Chilling words, and the harsh conditions which followed generalized a fear of 'the workhouse' which still persists in many old people's minds.

The Local Government Act of 1929 replaced the Boards of Guardians by local and county authorities. 1929 to 1948 was the heyday of the voluntary hospitals and the 'infirmaries' but these concentrated largely on acute medical conditions and by-passed old people except for the 'chronic sick' wards. With the advent of the Health Service in 1948 the workhouses were gradually taken over, at first often being jointly used as dormitories and (second rate) hospitals. The National Assistance Act of 1948, pioneered by Aneurin Bevan, put a statutory duty on the Local Authority to provide residential care for old people who could not manage to live at home.

The Social Services have steadily increased in both extent and variety since that time and, though still in many aspects quite inadequate, are of great importance to a large number of old people, many of whom could not survive independently in their own homes without the help offered.

## Organization

The Social Services and the Health Services are two independently operating branches of the Health and Social Services Division of the State Department of Health and Social Security. Figure 22.1 illustrates the broad structure of the organizations.

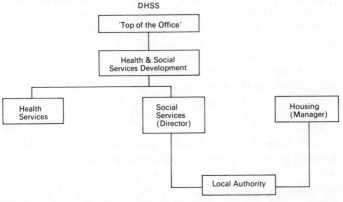

Fig. 22.1 Structure of social services: block diagram of broad organization structure.

The basic working unit of the Social Services is a Department, whose catchment area corresponds, not always accurately, with that of one or more Health Districts. The responsibility for setting up these SSD's lies with the Local Authority, usually a County Council or Metropolitan District, which also allocates the funds for maintenance and improvement of the services. The actual extent of provision therefore depends heavily on the political complexion and 'tradition' of the Local Authority: some are forward-looking and generous, others are blinkered in the tradition of sturdy self-dependence and are correspondingly mean.

The personal Social Services underwent a fundamental reorganization as a result of the 'Local Authority Social Services Act of 1970'. Before then, the SSD consisted of a number of specialist units—child health, mental welfare, etc. —and the officers concerned dealt with specialized casework. The act of 1970 aimed to provide a unified system of local authority services integrated in one Department, and the consequence for the field workers was that they were transformed more or less overnight into 'generic' social workers dealing with all the kinds of problems occurring in a family unit. Distant tremors from this earthquake are still felt but in general the organization has proved successful: in geriatric practice it promises to make easier the thorny task of coordinating services for old people discharged from hospital.

Where old people are concerned the new unified SSD's provide some or all of these facilities:

1. Residential accommodation ('old people's homes')
2. Home Help Service
3. 'Meals on Wheels'
4. Day Centres
5. Laundry service for incontinent people
6. Night attendants
7. Welfare facilities for the physically handicapped in general. These are often relevant to old people.

## Residential accommodation

Old People's Homes (often called 'Part III Homes' since they were dealt with in Part III of the Act of 1948 quoted above) are self-contained units in which old people can live out their last years in something which at least approaches a domestic atmosphere. Some are converted large, old houses: they suffer frequently from the disadvantage of having no elevator, but are often highly successful in a social sense. The great and increasing majority are, however, purpose-built units housing

30 to 40 people of both sexes, most of whom will have their own room and there are communal dining and sitting rooms. Though they are comfortable and convenient residences, not all old people find themselves happily at home in modern airport lounge style accommodation.

*Which old people qualify for admission?* There are no formally prescribed criteria for acceptance into a residential home. Obviously, with the present chronic shortage of places, only those genuinely incapable of self-care in their own homes will be admitted: mere preference for being 'looked after' in a home is not as yet a good enough reason, though it is hard to see why an old person who has struggled gallantly to remain independent but finds it no longer worth the candle, should not have a right of admission (as happens now in some parts of Scandinavia).

A minimum degree of competence in the 'activities of daily living' is necessary for residents in Old People's Homes: ideally they will be able to get in and out of a chair and bed unaided, to dress without help and to be mobile enough to get to the lavatory and dining room albeit with difficulty and slowly (if necessary in a self-propelling wheelchair). Many of these residents will, however, require some degree of assistance.

Two controversial aspects are the required degree of mental clarity and continence. About 16 per cent of all residents in Old People's Homes are confused, and in general they are well tolerated, except for two habits: nocturnal wandering into other residents' rooms and endless chattering. Probably many confused patients actually benefit from being in a relatively normal social framework, but there is clearly a limit to the number of confused patients who can be housed, without worsening the quality of life for the nonconfused resident. Frankly antisocial or aggressive behaviour will justifiably disqualify.

Some degree of urinary incontinence is also tolerable and rarely causes objections from the other residents. But regular nocturnal bed-wetting or faecal incontinence puts an enormous load on the staff: it is important to realize that most Homes do not have nursing-trained staff.

*Who decides about admission?* The Social Services Department have the complete right of decision about the placing of old people in such homes: the medical doctor may advise about his patient being admitted but cannot insist. Clearly the Social Services must balance the needs of old people needing admission direct from the community, against those of patients already in hospital.

The Social Services have a statutory duty to keep a register of all handicapped people in their area, and since old people constitute about 65 per cent of all the handicapped, many old people will be known to Social Services and their requirement for a place in a residential home foreseen.

*Who pays?* In general, the residents themselves contribute about half of the national cost of maintaining Old People's Homes. The rates are set by Parliament, but are adjusted according to the resident's financial means. Enough will always be left to meet small personal needs.

*Sheltered accommodation*

There are at present about 125 000 places in Old People's Homes in England and Wales: they accommodate only 1·7 per cent of the over 65 population. Although waiting lists are, as already commented long, expansion of this type of accommodation has always been slow, about 2·8 per cent increase per annum, and has recently slowed even further, in favour of a switch to 'sheltered accommodation' as a national policy.

There is no standard pattern for sheltered housing. Often it consists of a cluster of bungalows or low-rise flats occupied only by old people and in a quiet neighbourhood but near shops. Recent purpose-built blocks of flatlets, for either single or married people, are often of excellent quality and include a restaurant and communal sitting rooms in the complex.

Many of these sheltered units are supervised by a warden whose duty is confined to daily checks that all is well with the residents, either through an 'intercom' or by personal visit, and to call help when needed: their duties do not include shopping, domestic cleaning or personal services.

Residents in this type of accommodation must be reasonably self-sufficient, able to cook, clean and care to some extent for themselves, but they will very often depend heavily on the support of a Home Help.

## Home help service

The Home Help Service is a powerful prop of many old people. Home Helps are usually married women living near the old people they serve. The tasks undertaken normally include cleaning, tidying, lighting fires, washing up, shopping and bed-making, but some will also help with cooking and washing. Often a warm personal relationship is established between the old person and the Home Help, whose arrival may be the only social event of the day. But frequent switching of Home Helps to different clients often causes dissatisfaction.

The service is, with some honourable exceptions, charged to the old person, again according to his means. The cost depends on the length and frequency of the sessions given: most old people will have a Home Help once or twice weekly for 1 to 3 hours, but in real need a seven days a week service can be given.

In general this service is well organized and an enormous boon to many old people.

## Meals on wheels

Except in large metropolitan areas this service, which consists of a hot meal delivered at about midday, is given by voluntary organizations, the Women's Royal Voluntary Service the British Red Cross Society or Age Concern, (who can receive support from Social Services in the shape of staff, premises or equipment). In towns the SSD may operate its own scheme.

An old person will usually get one or two meals weekly: five times a week is less common and seven times rare and usually unnecessary. The service varies from one locality to another, as there is no statutory duty to provide these meals.

There is a charge of a few pence for each meal but the service is heavily subsidised from public funds.

## Day centres

Day centres are not part of the hospital service but are really clubs for old people. They provide meals, some kind of recreational activity and an opportunity for an old person to meet others. Arrangements for attendance are made by hospitals, family doctors or social workers. Separate day centres are mostly found in large towns but some local authorities are now accepting old people into Part 3 homes for day care. Loneliness being as prevalent as it is among old people, the Day Centres serve a useful function.

They are not, however, a place for management of the physically sick: this is the role of the *Day Hospital* which conversely is not intended for use as a club. (see p. 223)

### Incontinence service

Some large towns (and almost no small ones) provide a service for incontinent patients and their relatives, in which soiled bed linen is taken away and returned clean. However, the delivery rarely occurs more than once a week, a period which is too long for the average household to tolerate accumulation of soiled linen. Customarily the service is given by the Local Authority. Rarely, linen is provided on loan. This is a useful service at present inadequate in scope. The patient is charged *pro rata* for the service.

The Home Help Organizer of the local SSD will provide information about the availability of a local incontinence service.

### Night attendants

This service provides someone (who is not usually a nurse) to look after infirm old folk during the evening or through the night. The main aim is to relieve the burden on caring relatives and give them a night off. The cost is charged to the old person but as with Home Helps, is adjustable. It is very patchy in distribution.

FURTHER READING

Willmott, Phyllis (1974) *Consumer's Guide to the British Social Services.* 4th edition. Penguin: Harmondsworth.

# 23. Voluntary Services

Volunteers have always played an important part in Great Britain towards making life easier for underprivileged groups and a great deal of voluntary activity is directed both to old people in their own homes and also to old people in hospital. The major organization concerned with this type of care is Age Concern which began in 1940 as the National Old People's Welfare Committee and subsequently became the National Old People's Welfare Council. Throughout the 35 years of its life, this movement has sponsored the development of almost 12 000 local committees throughout Great Britain, each of which in turn has been responsible for the development of old peoples' clubs, the organization of friendly visitors for isolated old people at home and in some cases for the provision of meals on wheels. These are the major and most important voluntary services provided in the community, but Age Concern organizations undertake and organize a host of other activities. These include the arrangement of holidays for old people, help with gardening and house decorating, the provision of organized 'good neighbour' services, the provision of Day Centres and of special transport to take old people both to Day Centres and also to visit their relatives in hospital, and so on. Where the local Age Concern committees are strong, as in many of the counties and larger towns, they act as a co-ordinating body for all services for the elderly and representatives of the various voluntary services meet with representatives of the hospital geriatric service, social services, housing departments and education departments, to discuss together the needs of old people in their area and particularly the contribution that can be made by volunteer groups.

Age Concern England (and its counterparts in Scotland, Wales and Northern Ireland) is also a body involved in social action and the promotion of old people's welfare at a national level. It has commissioned much research both into its own activities (e.g. voluntary visiting, day care, special housing for the elderly, etc.) and also into the wider needs and aspirations of old people (e.g. the problems of heating, the special problems of minority groups such as, aging immigrants, and the rights of old people in institutions, etc.). Age Concern collates information of all types concerned with elderly people and with aging and distributes this widely. It provides training courses for volunteers as well as for workers in various types of health and social care and it speaks for the elderly on a national scale about their needs and problems.

It publishes a national journal *Age Concern Today*.

Another important voluntary organization in Great Britain is the *Pre-retirement Association*. This is a national organization which has a network of local branches. Its objective is to organize and develop day release classes for workers in industry where they may have the opportunity to consider the implications of retirement for themselves and to prepare for it while they are still in employment. Pre-retirement courses of this type are held in many adult education centres, usually with the workers being seconded one day a week for six, eight or ten weeks, ideally five to ten years before they retire. The implications of retirement which are discussed include finance, housing, retirement migration to the seaside, health, the importance of maintaining a routine, and creative or recreational interests, and the possibilities for work, paid or unpaid, after retirement.

The Pre-retirement Association publishes a monthly journal called *Choice*.

*Voluntary work in hospitals*

Many hospitals now employ a full time co-ordinator of voluntary services whose responsibility it is to recruit volunteers and to deploy them throughout the hospital in areas where their services are most needed and in work which they will enjoy doing. Many of these organizers have been extremely successful in their work which is of particular importance in relation to long-stay patients in both geriatric and psychiatric wards.

# 24. Care of the Dying

*'A time to live and a time to die'*

Medical education and practice rightly lay their great emphasis on the preservation of life. The student must learn and the physician must realize, however, that because a medical or surgical procedure is possible it is not necessarily right and the doctor who cannot see that there is a human being inside a tangle of clinical problems is not the person to look after dying patients.

It is important, therefore, that the emphasis on preservation of life should not blunt the doctor's sensitivity to care of dying people and particularly should not make him see death as failure. This unconscious feeling may impose a barrier between the doctor and the sympathetic care of his dying patient. He may feel he has nothing to offer and is therefore embarrassed and as a result quickly passes by the bed of the terminally ill patient. There is a danger also that he may rationalize that the patient is unable to bear the truth. The result of all this may be that contacts between the doctor and his patient centre on trivialities and untruths and prevent the dying patient from obtaining the help and support which he might expect from his physician.

This sad state of affairs was highlighted in a symposium on 'Care of the Dying' held in the Royal College of Physicians in 1972. The opening speaker, the actress Sheila Hancock, said that when she was told that her mother had cancer and the prognosis was poor. 'The awful thing that I found was that there was nowhere that I could turn for comfort and help. What I did find again and again (and this is a generalization) was an attitude in the medical profession of appearing not to want to know about the incurably ill.'

In many ways death in old age is of a different quality to the death of younger people. It is less often due to malignant disease and is more often preceded by a period of coma. Above all, most people dying in old age have come to terms with the fact that life is finite and are prepared to die. Death in younger people often seems more unjust and may be more of a tragedy for those who are left behind.

The following discussion is not concerned exclusively with death in old age. The management of dying patients and care of their relatives is an important part of the education of all doctors.

It is sometimes said that death has replaced sex as a taboo subject in late twentieth century western society. There is no doubt that the personal experience of close contact with a dying person is no longer the universal experience of people in the first half of their lives. If a death occurs at home there is a tendency to shield children from it and to send them away at the time of the funeral so that they do not experience the understanding of death and of bereavement which can only come from personal involvement. It is noteworthy that Sheila Hancock in the address referred to above indicates that she had reached middle age without having any first-hand experience of death whatsoever. The fact that about two thirds of deaths occur in hospital and that bodies are laid out in funeral parlours rather than in patients' homes is another change in the behaviour of our society which keeps death a remote experience.

Fortunately, there is evidence of increasing awareness among doctors and nurses of the important role which they may play in relation to death and dying and it is to be hoped that this will be followed by a change in the attitude of our society towards death and the bereavement.

## The mental aspects of dying

An American psychiatrist, Dr Kubler-Ross, in her book *On Death and Dying* divides the dying process into four stages. The first is the stage of *denial*: 'No not me, it cannot be true'. She believes this is an almost universal reaction and emphasizes how important it is for doctors and nurses to respect the patient's wishes in allowing this stage to continue as long as may be required; a period which may vary from a few hours to many months. It will pass and will be replaced by partial acceptance.

The second stage is that of *anger:* 'Why me?' This anger may be projected to all members of the staff and of the patient's family. It is a difficult stage to handle and it is important that the attendant should understand the reason for the anger and not take it personally.

The third stage is that of *bargaining*. The fact is accepted, but the patient tries to obtain certain promises (from God and from the staff). It may be that she will live long enough to attend her daughter's wedding (although the real object is to prolong life). These promises may be associated with guilt and the doctor should not brush them aside lightly.

The fourth stage is one of *depression*. The depression may be twofold, partly induced by loss suffered already (for instance, as a result of mastectomy or hysterectomy), but more importantly the losses which are pending. This depression may be suffered silently and patients should be encouraged to express their sorrow and certainly not be told to 'look on the bright side'.

The final stage is one of *acceptance* and it is particularly important that this should not be disturbed by ill-advised last-ditch surgical procedures attempting to snatch a few more weeks of life. The period of acceptance leading to death is one characterized by sleep and a diminished wish for verbal communication. It should not be mistaken for a happy stage. It is a stage almost void of feelings. The patient wishes to be left alone more and it is the family who now increasingly require the doctor's support.

All those who are especially involved in care of dying patients emphasize that the doctor's role in relation to these mental attributes is to be prepared to listen, to share realities with the patient whenever possible but not to force on him abrupt statements about prognosis. In particular, patients should never be told that they have 'X' number of years to live. If doctors will listen they can usually guide their patients into a real acceptance of their situation without either maintaining an unreal charade on the one hand or being unfeelingly brusque on the other.

Patients often pick up clues about their real situation from all that is going on around them. If they wish to talk about these things the doctors and nurses should make time to listen to them. At the very end a physical presence for a little while, a period of non-verbal communication, is what is needed and reassurances can be conveyed by facial expression and hand pressure.

While most dying patients wish to come to a realization of their situation, albeit in their own time, most will also wish to cling to some vestige of hope however unreal. When the situation is acknowledged, therefore, the doctor should make it quite clear that while there is nothing else that he can do to remove the pathological process, he will nevertheless continue to do all that is possible to relieve symptoms and prevent distress.

## Physical attributes

In old age dying is frequently preceded by *immobility, incontinence* and *mental abnormality*. Isaacs discovered that 40 per cent of those aged 65 and over dying in Glasgow had one or more of these three disabilities lasting for a month prior to death and that 20 per cent had one or more of them lasting for a year prior to death. These indicate, of course, the burden which has to be carried by relatives and that these are important reasons why old people are admitted to hospital for their period of dying. Exton-Smith has indicated that symptoms of physical discomfort occurred in about one fifth of elderly people dying in hospital, 14 per cent suffering moderate or severe pain and 8 per cent other distressing symptoms, particularly respiratory distress and nausea and vomiting. It is the doctor's rôle to alleviate these symptoms. The control of pain is a paramount responsibility and the armamentarium of analgesic drugs now available will allow this to be done with complete effectiveness in the majority of cases. Occasionally intractable pain requires a neurosurgical approach to cut the pain-carrying tracts within the spinal cord.

Select an adequate analgesic. It is the doctor's responsibility to ensure that consecutive doses are given to anticipate the recurrence of pain. Analgesics should not be given mechanically on a four or six hourly basis so that patients have to wait in pain until the next dose is due. The right dose/time interval has to be 'titrated' in each case to prevent the emergence of pain. By this means the total amount of analgesic needed in the long run is often less than with more infrequent or haphazard administration. It should be emphasized once again that the distress of pain in dying should no longer be suffered by patients.

Simple analgesics should be used to begin with including aspirin, paracetamol, methadone, dihydrocodeine or nepenthe. Later, opiates should be introduced. Probably the most effective of all is diamorphine which is very often given in a mixture with cocaine (the 'Brompton Mixture') and sometimes with the addition of alcohol (the 'Brompton Cocktail'). These have the advantage that they can be taken by mouth. Sometimes their effect can be potentiated by a small dose of a phenothiazine given to diminish anxiety.

Pain many of course be due to complications such as pneumonia, or a pathological fracture, or urinary infection. The use of surgery or antibiotics may be indicated in these cases to relieve the pain.

Useful in the control of nausea and vomiting are cyclizine metaclopramide and prochlorperazine. Unfortunately, the relief of respiratory distress is not so easy.

## Where to die

Of all deaths in this country about two thirds occur in hospital and the remainder at home and the trend all the time is towards increasing hospital admission for dying patients. In old age increasing numbers of patients die in hospital and Isaacs showed that in Glasgow every women over 85 spent an average of the last six months of her life in hospital. It is probably true that most patients would prefer to die at home if facilities were available for their care and if they did not feel that they were being a burden to their relatives. Whenever possible, therefore, domiciliary services should be mobilized to make it possible for the dying person to stay in his own familiar environment where his individual personal needs are much more likely to be acceded to.

In hospital, patients may be admitted to any of a whole variety of wards and it is probably best that those who have had investigations and treatment in a surgical or medical ward and have come to know and trust the staff should be readmitted to that ward should hospitalization be necessary at the end of their lives. A number of special hospitals or hospices for care of dying patients have been created in the last 25 years, some by religious organizations and some secular. They usually attempt to admit patients only with a prognosis less than three months; they generally have some beds which are financed by the National Health Service, and others which are supported by charity. Perhaps the best known of all is St Christopher's Hospice in South London.

These hospices or hospitals for the dying are not the forbidding places which they may sound, since they are usually bright and sunny and staffed by doctors and nurses who are specially skilled in the management of dying patients. The staff are trained to listen and they are experts in the pharmacological management of dying. They aim to involve the family from the beginning and their success is apparent to all who have had contact with them.

The question that arises is, to what extent should special hospices and hospitals for the dying be created? It seems unlikely, in general, that they can be any more than a limited number of centres of excellence, used for teaching as well as for care, and pointing the way for others to follow.

## Bereavement

Care of the dying inevitably moves to care of the bereaved and there is great advantage if continuity of care can be maintained for both the dying patient and for his surviving relatives. Bereavement is a period of grieving and the expression of grief would seem to be an essential process for the bereaved. Doctors should see, therefore, that bereaved relatives have the opportunity to go through the stages of the process of grieving. These are likely to be at first a stage of numbness, followed by weeping and sobbing and then a stage of depression. It is generally best to allow patients to live through these stages and not to try and short circuit them unless they appear interminable. In old age the depression following bereavement may not be self-limiting and there is, therefore, a time when treatment may be needed. This may involve simple encouragement to socialize or it may require treatment with antidepressant drugs or psychiatric management.

On the death of a spouse an old person may find that the loss of pension means that he is less well-off and important decisions may have to be taken as to whether he will remain alone, move in with relatives or apply for some other form of care. These decisions should not be taken precipitately and certainly not within the first few weeks of bereavement. No irrevocable decisions of this type should be made until the main period of grieving has passed.

## Euthanasia

Euthanasia is a topic of public discussion and has been the subject of Parliamentary Bills although these have not been successful and euthanasia is illegal. However, it is important that doctors should know what is meant by euthanasia and consider its implications since they will almost certainly be asked to express an opinion about it from time to time.

The first important matter is to discover a definition of euthanasia. This may be best understood as the deliberate termination of life under carefully defined conditions (with legal agreement, being carried out in the presence of witnesses and with the agreement of relatives). The essential element, however, is that of request, and euthanasia has been defined by Professor Dunstan as 'homicide upon request'. Dunstan distinguishes it carefully from suicide (which is not illegal) assisted suicide (which is a crime) and other methods of life termination which he describes as senicide or dementicide (that is the killing of aged and of demented people) or amenticide. None of these is what is understood as euthanasia and all of them are crimes. It should be emphasized also that euthanasia is not the acceleration of death as the result of side-effects of drugs used for the relief of intractable pain, for in this case the drug is used with the intention of killing pain. Nor is it about the deliberate withholding of an antibiotic or other technical or surgical procedures which might have the effect of temporarily prolonging the dying patient's life.

By euthanasia then is meant the bringing about of a patient's death at his request and there is no doubt that whatever minority views there may be about the desirability of legalizing such a procedure it is not supported by doctors. A survey carried out by the medical staff of a large teaching hospital showed only 2 per cent in sympathy with the aims of legalized euthanasia.

The basic reasons for this are on moral grounds but it is worth recalling that there are a number of practical implications of euthanasia as well: for instance, there are the interests of the patient's relatives who in an emotionally charged situation are likely to have 'ambivalent feelings of attachment and of wanting to be free' (Dunstan) and who may also have material and financial interests relating to the patient's death. Of equal and perhaps greater importance, would be the breach of trust likely to be created between patients and physician or nurse when 'the needle or the draft in a nurse's hand could not be accepted assurably as a vehicle of comfort if not of healing, but might be—might be—an instrument of death' (Dunstan). Doctors and nurses may thus become a target not only of suspicion but also of possible litigation.

FURTHER READING

Department of Health and Social Security (1973) *Reports on Health and Social Subjects*, volume 5, *Care of the Dying*. London: HMSO.
Hinton, J. (1972) *Dying*. London: Penguin.
Kubler-Ross, E. (1970) *On Death and Dying*. London: Tavistock Publications.

# 25. Some Legal Aspects of Geriatric Care

## Patients in hospital unable to manage their own affairs

It often happens that an elderly patient—often a widow or widower without any surviving children—is believed, after assessment in hospital, to be incapable of ever returning home to lead an independent existance. Two familiar practical problems in this connexion are:

1. The patient lives in accommodation which is rented in his or her name either from a Local Authority or from a private person, and contains personal effects

2. The patient owns a house or other property or has substantial investments.

*Patient living in rented property.* The National Assistance Act of 1947, Section 48, puts a duty on the local council (of the area in which the patient's *property* is situated, not the patient) to take suitable measures to care for the property and goods of patients in hospital. Information on which the council will act is usually gathered in the hospital concerned by the Medical Social Worker, who tells it to the Local Authority Social Services Department's 'Assessment Section'.

If it is a simple, small scale matter as in (1), the Social Services Department will first ask the medical attendant in hospital to certify in writing (there is no standard national form) that the patient is unable to manage her affairs, is very unlikely to return home and that it would be in the patient's best interests for the tenancy to be terminated and her effects sold. The action required will be taken by a relative if one can be found who is willing to do so: if none can be found the Social Services Department will make the arrangements. Money from the sale of the patient's property or goods will usually be paid to the patient's account with the hospital's Finance Officer.

2. *A patient with substantial property unable to manage his or*

*her affairs.* If a patient owns a house or has investments, rents, trusts etc. the matter is more complicated and here the Court of Protection will probably be invoked.

*The Court of Protection* exists specifically to protect and control the administration of the property and affairs of persons who, through mental disorder, are incapable of managing their own affairs. Its work applies to people of all ages, but is of special relevance to old people because of their high prevalence of mental confusion.

The address of the Court (which is not a 'Court' in the ordinary sense of the word, but the title of an office) is: Staffordshire House, 25 Store Street, London WC1. Full information on its practice and working is contained in the reference work by Heywood and Massey (1961) *Court of Protection Practice,* 8th edition, published by Stevens and Sons, Ltd.

The Court will consider taking over the administration of a patient's affairs only if a properly completed 'Originating Application' is made to it: it is unlikely to do so if a doctor in hospital writes an ordinary letter saying that a patient is unable to manage her affairs without giving a specific reason why management by the Court would seem necessary.

The 'Originating Application' is almost always drawn up and submitted by a solicitor, usually under instruction from a relative, or by the legal branch of a Local Authority. Personal Applications can, however, be made direct to the Court and the Official Solicitor of the Court can also originate an application.

The person in whose name the 'Originating Application' is made is almost always the nearest of the relatives if there be any. This should be the husband or wife, if alive, and if they are alive but do not originate the application, a reason has to be given. If there is no spouse, the nearest relative can choose to originate, and in the event of there being no relatives, a friend or even a creditor or debtor may apply. If there is conflict about the best originator, the Court will choose; the nearest of kin will be preferred, or the person 'most likely to bring out the whole truth'.

The patient's (hospital) doctor will be involved in this Originating Application only to the extent of being required.

on request to provide for the purpose either a 'Medical Affidavit' on the Court's Form CP2 for ordinary cases, or a 'Medical Certificate' Form CP3 in 'small property' cases. This form requests information on, *inter alia*, the medical reasons why a patient is believed incapable of managing his or her affairs, whether the surroundings can be appreciated etc. In cases of gross dementia the evidence is usually plentiful and unequivocal, but there may be real doubt, in which case the doctor is wise to get the support of a senior colleague experienced in such decisions, or the opinion of a psychiatrist.

The papers, including the doctor's Affidavit or certificate, are seen by the Court and the next step is that the patient is served with 'Notice of Originating Proceedings' (he is not served with a copy of the 'Originating Application'). The Court can dispense with Service of this Notice if it is satisfied that the patient is incapable of understanding the notice, but it rarely does so. The Notice must be seen by the patient without delay. Proof that he has been served with the Notice usually falls to the lot of the hospital doctor who is required to complete form CP7 which certifies that the patient has seen the notice. This may entail futile attempts to explain a legal document to a profoundly demented or aphasic patient who clearly cannot comprehend it at all. The simplest way is to explain this state of affairs on form CP7. The patient has, however, a legal right to object within seven days (in writing only) to the Court; this he can do himself or instruct a solicitor. The patient can contest the view that he is not fit to manage his affairs, he can object to the proposed 'Receiver', or give his view of how the property should be managed. On receiving his objection the Court may (1) make no order i.e. the Court will not be involved (2) proceed with the Order on the Master's discretion, if the patient seems unequivocally unable to manage his affairs, or (3) if there is doubt, the Master will ask for the Lord Chancellor's Medical Visitors to report on the patient's mental condition and advise about his capacity.

If there is no objection and proceedings continue, the Court will appoint a Receiver, but this and subsequent management do not involve the medical attendant.

The Court of Protection should not be confused with 'Power of Attorney' in which a person of sound mind voluntarily gives to someone else legal responsibility for the management of his financial affairs and estate, either generally or for some specific act. Verbal delegation is not enough and a legally prescribed 'Letter of Attorney' is drawn up by a solicitor.

## Patients admitted under an Order for their own care and protection

It happens, fortunately rarely, that a patient with gross physical or mental disease is believed by his medical attendant (either the family doctor or hospital doctor) to be in imperative need of hospital treatment because either the patient's own life or the life and health of others would otherwise be threatened. The patient may, however, refuse to co-operate. Admission to hospital or other public institution can then be compelled through Section 47 of the Public Assistance Act (1947) by an order of a Magistrates Court made on evidence submitted to the Local Health Authority, with the advice of the District Community Physician (to whom the family doctor or hospital doctor should first apply with an account of the case).

Where old people are concerned, the type of patient involved is often a recluse, living alone in squalid conditions and sometimes suffering from malnutrition or a disabling physical condition. Almost always there is a large mental element, though this will often not amount to a frank psychosis. 'Senile breakdown in standards of hygiene and cleanliness' is a syndrome which often raises the possibility of compulsory admission of an old person.

Often the neighbours will indignantly demand the patient's removal, fearful for their own safety, and on occasion with good reason, since some socially isolated old people are accident-prone, especially where fire is concerned.

The 'Order' lasts 48 hours only, but can be renewed. Sometimes a brief period of treatment and rehabilitation is enough to allow the patient to go home, especially if he can go to live with relatives, but often removal to hospital will shatter permanently his ability to survive (however unsatisfactorily) in the community. For this reason, compulsory admission under Section 47 should be avoided whenever possible.

# Index

# LIVINGSTONE MEDICAL TEXTS